Nutritarian Handbook
& NUTRIENT IQ FOOD SCORING GUIDE

OTHER BOOKS BY
Joel Fuhrman, M.D.

Eat For Life–
The Breakthrough Nutrient-Rich Program For Longevity, Disease Reversal
and Sustained WeightLoss

Eat to Live–
The Revolutionary Formula for Fast and Sustained Weight Loss

The End of Dieting–
Explores the Science of Nutrition and Provides a Simple and Effective Strategy
to Help you Lose Weight, Get Healthy and Stop Dieting

End of Diabetes–
The Eat to Live Plan to Prevent and Reverse Diabetes

End of Heart Disease–
The Eat to Live Plan to Prevent and Reverse Heart Disease

Super Immunity–
The Essential Guide for Boosting Your Body's Defenses
to Live Longer, Stronger, and Disease Free

The Eat to Live Cookbook–
Over 180 Nutrient-Rich Recipes
Plus Cooking and Food Purchasing Tips

The Eat to Live Quick & Easy Cookbook–
Over 131 Quick and Easy Nutritarian Recipes for Delicious Entrees, Salads,
Wraps, Dips, Dressings, Desserts and More

Fast Food Genocide–
How Processed Food Is Killing Us And What We Can Do About It

www.DrFuhrman.com
Dr. Fuhrman's official website for information,
recipes, supportive services, and products

Heal your body and transform your life at Dr. Fuhrman's

EAT TO LIVE RETREAT
San Diego County, California

At the Eat to Live Retreat, Dr. Fuhrman and his expert team will help you take control of your health. Drawing on his 30 years' experience practicing lifestyle medicine, Dr. Fuhrman will design a plan that will help you lose excess weight, reverse chronic disease, reduce / eliminate medications, and end addictive food behaviors.

This immersive experience includes delicious and organic Nutritarian meals prepared by expert chefs, cooking classes with our chefs, nutrition classes led by Dr. Fuhrman, group fitness classes that are individualized based on a person's strength and balance, group therapy sessions to discuss emotional eating and food addiction, aerobics in our salt water pool, and more. Our entire staff, including our house manager and full-time nurse, make sure your stay is a life-changing experience. You will go home with the knowledge and strategies to continue your journey to a healthy, long and vibrant life.

Find out more about this beautiful residential facility, located just 30 minutes north of downtown San Diego, by visiting DrFuhrman.com/etlretreat or call (949) 432-6295.

Nutritarian Handbook
& NUTRIENT IQ FOOD SCORING GUIDE

JOEL FUHRMAN, M.D.

PUBLISHED BY

Gift of Health Press

Contact:
Gift of Health Press
Flemington, NJ 08822
for wholesale inquiries go to:
giftofhealthpress.com

Printed in the United States of America
ISBN-13: 978-0-9992235-5-0
Library of Congress Control Number: 2011941079

Publisher's Note:
Do not start, stop, or change medication without professional medical
advice, and do not change your diet if you are ill or on medication,
except under the supervision of a competent physician. Neither this,
nor any other book, is intended to take the place of personalized
medical care or treatment.

ᏡᏢ
Gift of Health Press

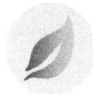

CONTENTS

INTRODUCTION

No one wants to have a heart attack, suffer a debilitating stroke or develop cancer. But lots of people die – unnecessarily – from these conditions every day. Nutritional science has made dramatic advances in recent years. The overwhelming accumulation of scientific knowledge points to a dramatic conclusion: The majority of diseases plaguing Americans are preventable. Using the information compiled from scientific studies, it is now possible to formulate a few simple diet and lifestyle principles that can save you years of suffering and premature death.

You have an opportunity that is unprecedented in human history: to enjoy better health and live longer than ever before. But being in the best of health and living longer comes at a price. How much would it be worth to you for a guarantee that you would never have a heart attack or a stroke? What would it be worth to you to healthfully and happily watch your children and grandchildren grow?

What would you be willing to pay for the assurance that you would not leave your spouse or your children all alone? Fortunately, the expenditure is infinitely affordable – little more than the effort needed to establish new, more healthful eating habits.

Everything in this book is supported by the preponderance of evidence from scientific studies. Still, the facts and guidelines will astound most physicians. Although the research is readily available for all to see, most people still have no idea that food can be the most powerful weapon in the fight against the major illnesses that plague our society. Now is the time for you to open your eyes to the value of superior nutrition, put wholesome food in your body, and take control of your health destiny.

CHAPTER ONE

AMERICA'S HEALTH CRISIS AND YOU

Americans are digging their graves with their knives and forks. It is not news that Americans are sickly and fat; almost everybody knows modern America is in the midst of an all-you-can eat food fest that has us literally bursting at the seams. We are not only eating ourselves into sickness and premature death, but we also have a health care crisis with upward-spiraling medical care costs. The economic costs of heart disease and other diet-related chronic diseases are staggering. In 1970, health care spending in the United States totaled $74.6 billion. By 2000, total health expenditures had reached about $1.4 trillion; in 2017, the amount spent had more than doubled to $3.5 trillion.[1]

Excess fat is detrimental at any level. Health care costs increase in parallel with body mass measurements, even beginning at the recommended body weights.[3]

In other words, health care costs start to rise even for the mildly overweight. These out-of-control costs play an important role in business failures, bankruptcies and loss of jobs. Our health system relies on an ever-expanding arsenal of medications, tests and procedures that fail to address the root cause of our escalating ill health: the way we choose to eat and live. In America, we have attempted to solve our dietary-caused health woes with the development of multiple medications for diabetes, hypertension and cholesterol-lowering. We have relied on heart procedures and surgeries, all at a dramatic expense with little benefit. We have been led to believe that drugs and doctors save lives, but the statistics show otherwise – lifespan is not significantly enhanced by the vast majority of medical interventions.

The Obesity Epidemic

Nutritionally caused disease is now the largest cause of death throughout the world. For the first time, the number of overweight individuals exceeds the number of those who are underweight. In recent years, the growth of processed foods, convenience foods and fast foods has supplied our relatively sedentary society with a diet of high-calorie foods with few nutrients. In all parts of the world, obesity appears to escalate as income increases and fast food and processed foods become available. Nowhere has this problem become as large as in America, where we have the biggest waistlines in the world. In the United States, being overweight is the norm, and almost all adults eventually take medications for their heart, diabetes, cholesterol or blood pressure. The number of obese Americans is higher than the number of those who smoke, use illegal drugs or suffer from other physical ailments. Obesity is a major risk factor associated with highly prevalent and serious diseases, such as heart disease, cancer and diabetes. The diet-style that creates these diseases fuels out-of-control medical costs. Seventy-one percent of Americans today are overweight or obese, up from 45 percent in 1960.[4] The average American today weighs almost 30 pounds more than they did 60 years ago, and has a considerably higher risk of heart attack, stroke and cancer to show for it.

Health Complications of Obesity

- Increased overall mortality
- Adult-onset diabetes
- Hypertension
- Degenerative arthritis
- Coronary artery disease
- Obstructive sleep apnea
- Gallstones
- Fatty infiltration of liver
- Restrictive lung disease
- Cancer

Poor Nutrition Everywhere

In the 20th century, processed foods became increasingly prevalent in the average American diet.

The consumption of fresh produce and whole grains plummeted, while the consumption of animal products increased. As a result, Americans now consume far more calories, fat, cholesterol, refined sugar, animal protein, sodium, and white flour, and far less fiber and plant-derived nutrients than is healthful. Obesity, diabetes, heart disease and cancer have skyrocketed.

CHANGE IN FOOD CONSUMPTION IN THE LAST 100 YEARS IN THE UNITED STATES

	1900	2000
Sugar	5 lbs/year	170 lbs/year
Soft drinks	0	53 gallons/year
Oils	4 lbs/year	74 lbs/year
Cheese	2 lbs/year	30 lbs/year
Meat	140 lbs/year	200 lbs/year
Homegrown Produce	131 lbs/year	11 pounds/year
Calories	2100/day	2757/day

Our society has evolved to a level of economic sophistication that allows us to eat ourselves to death. A diet centered on milk, cheese, pasta, bread, fried foods, sugar-filled snacks, and drinks lays the groundwork for obesity, cancer, heart disease, diabetes and autoimmune illnesses. It is not solely that these foods are harmful; it is also what we are not eating that is causing the problem. We are not eating enough nutrient-rich produce.

When you calculate all the calories consumed from the Standard American Diet, you find that the calories coming from the most health-promoting foods, such as fresh fruit, vegetables (not including white potatoes), beans, raw nuts, and seeds, are less than 10 percent of the total caloric intake. This dangerously low intake of unrefined plant foods is what guarantees weakened immunity to infectious disease, frequent illnesses and a shorter lifespan. We will never win the war on cancer, heart disease, diabetes, and other degenerative illnesses unless we address this deficiency. Though the American diet has spread all over the world, bringing with it heart disease, cancer and obesity, studies still show that in the populations that eat more fruits and vegetables, the incidences of death from these diseases is dramatically lowered.

COMPOSITION OF THE AMERICAN DIET

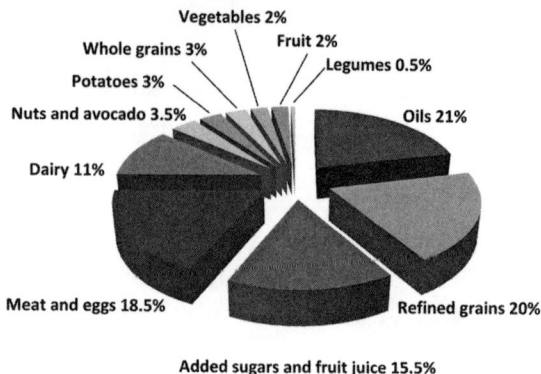

Vegetables 2%

Fruit 2%

Whole grains 3%

Legumes 0.5%

Potatoes 3%

Nuts and avocado 3.5%

Oils 21%

Dairy 11%

Meat and eggs 18.5%

Refined grains 20%

Added sugars and fruit juice 15.5%

United States Department of Agriculture. Economic Research Service. Food Availability (Per Capita) Data System [https://www.ers.usda.gov/data-products/food-availability-per-capita-data-system/food-availability-per-capita-data-system/]

Heart Disease is Preventable

Heart disease is a much bigger problem than most people think. It is the leading cause of death for both men and women in the United States. It affects almost all Americans, with one in four adults taking prescription cholesterol-lowering medication.[5] Yet heart disease is one of the top preventable causes of death. Modern medical techniques and drugs cannot win this war, because the true cause of disease is overlooked. Heart disease, and most other common modern diseases are caused by inadequate nutrition. The tragedy is enormous. When you consider that nobody really has to die from a heart- or circulatory system-related death, it is even more of a tragedy. The disability, suffering and years of life lost are almost totally the result of dietary ignorance. It is not impossible or even difficult to protect yourself; you simply must eat properly. Nothing else can offer such dramatic protection.

DEATHS FROM DISEASES OF THE HEART

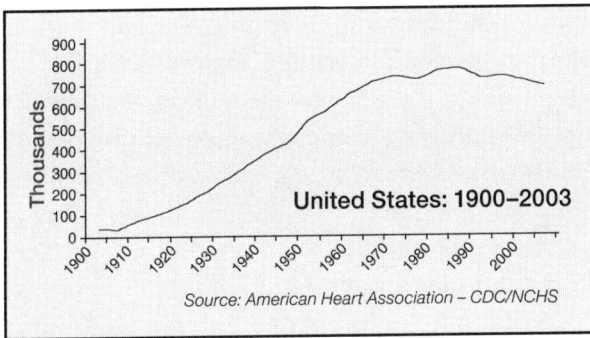

Source: American Heart Association – CDC/NCHS

Four Simple Truths
While America's health crisis is real, you can reclaim your health. Consider these four critical points:

- We are brainwashed into thinking that drugs are the answer to our health problems

- Unhealthy food is addictive

- Foods that don't contain health-promoting micronutrients lead to overeating

• A normal body weight in conjunction with nutritional adequacy is essential for good health and longevity

Understanding these simple truths is the key to solving the health care problems of most Americans. The cells in our bodies need a wide array of nutrients, numbering in the thousands, to function normally. The human body is designed to be fueled by natural, nutrient-rich plant food. Foods supply not just vitamins and minerals, but thousands of immune-supporting substances called phytochemicals that are essential for our protection against disease. While science has described these needs, an astonishing 95 percent of Americans do not even meet the Center for Disease Control's (CDC's) minimum nutritional guidelines for all the basic vitamins and minerals.[6] Very few people eat healthfully enough to protect themselves against disease in later life.

Why Diets Fail

Low-nutrient eating drives overeating behavior and is the primary cause of obesity, disease and death in the modern world. Have you ever been on a diet, losing and gaining the same 10, 20 or 30 pounds? The number of people who successfully lose weight through dieting and keep it off for the rest of their lives is fewer than two out of 100.[7] More than 98 percent of people who lose weight gain it back, which is often unhealthier than not losing it at all. Only the right information and the proper tools will give you permanent results.

The biggest problem with most diets is that you are asked to deprive yourself, using portion control, low carbs, fewer calories, etc. Deprivation never works, and your food cravings return with a vengeance! This is the basis of the "yo-yo" dieting industry. I want you to know that it's not that you have failed a diet; it's that the system (diets, magic pills, surgeries, etc.) has failed you. My findings, based on my 30 years of experience with over 10,000 patients, and thousands of supportive research studies, is that a properly nourished body will seek its ideal weight. So instead of "dieting," I want to show you the foods that provide the nutrition your body needs. The body has an incredible ability to heal itself and get back in balance when you feed it what it needs. It's that simple! Your body is like a supercomputer: Feed it right, and it will keep you fit, lean and healthy.

Enjoy a Full, More Pleasurable Life

If you are reading this, it is likely that you are someone who is ready to take control of your health. Superior nutrition is the foundation of this diet. It is the path to medical wellness in your life. It is the most powerful intervention, not only to prevent disease, but to also reverse it. Complete recovery from most chronic degenerative illnesses is possible.

The information presented here is the fastest and most effective way to create an optimal nutritional environment for self-healing. This plant-based, high-nutrient dense diet can enable you to avoid angioplasty, bypass surgery and other invasive procedures. By adopting this eating style, you can protect yourself against heart attack, stroke and dementia. You can reduce and eventually eliminate your need for prescription drugs. You will not only optimize your health and potentially save your life; this eating style will also increase the pleasure you get from food.

It will result in the lessening of hunger, the removal of addiction, and – if needed – profound and long-term weight loss. I have seen this in my medical practice and it has been documented in medical publications.[8] You will not only reach your ideal body weight, but you will enjoy a longer, more healthful and pleasurable life. More and more, new medical studies are investigating and demonstrating that diets rich in high-nutrient plant foods have a suppressive effect on appetite and are most effective for long-term weight control.[9] The healthiest way to eat is also the most successful way to obtain a favorable weight, if you consider long-term results.

I am thrilled to be able to work with you and address your diet-related health issues. You will learn how to feed your body so it operates at its highest level every day. Your energy levels will be amazing, without relying on artificial stimulants like coffee and sugar. You will sleep better, your skin will look better and you will feel and look younger. In short, your properly nourished body will allow you to live life to the fullest!

I encourage you to read my books, *Eat for Life*, *The End of Dieting*, *The End of Heart Disease*, *The End of Diabetes* and *Super Immunity* for a more comprehensive understanding and application of these principles. I also offer an assortment of valuable membership features at DrFuhrman.com, where you can obtain more detailed and personalized health and nutritional guidance.

My **Eat to Live Retreat** in San Diego County California is open year round to help you resolve your medical issues, and give you the additional support you need to reach and maintain your ideal weight.

CHAPTER TWO

BECOMING A NUTRITARIAN

Not Your Typical Diet

Typical diet books usually contain a list of rules and regulations to restrict calories for weight loss. This is a problem, because when the focus is weight loss alone, results are rarely permanent.

The focus in this handbook is on nutrition and eating healthfully, which is an undisputed, yet often overlooked critical ingredient for any dietary success. Here, there is no carbohydrate, protein or calorie counting, portion-size measuring or weighing involved. In fact, you will eat substantial, satisfying portions amount of food, and still, over time, you will become healthier and will be satisfied with fewer calories. A properly nourished body will automatically seek its ideal weight, without having to fight the scale or count calories.

The fundamentals of this eating style are to increase high-nutrient foods in your diet and to "crowd out" unhealthful, low-nutrient foods. What does it mean to "crowd out"? It means that as you eat more delicious, high-nutrient foods, you will be reducing your desire for fatty, processed and unhealthful products. The major tenet of the Nutritarian diet is: moderate caloric restriction in the context of micronutrient excellence. That means taking in sufficient micronutrients without consuming excess calories.

When you change the foods you eat to better meet your nutrient needs, you feel better and it eventually becomes your preferred way of eating. To accomplish this, you will be presented with scientific, logical information that explains the connection between food and your weight and health. If you need to lose weight, this information will help you shed pounds naturally and easily, merely as a side effect of eating so healthfully.

What is a Nutritarian?
When you learn and practice this eating style, you can proudly call yourself a Nutritarian. A Nutritarian is someone who strives to consume and learns to prefer foods that are nutritious. Quite simply, a Nutritarian:

- Eats mainly high-nutrient, natural plant foods: vegetables, fruits, beans, nuts and seeds.

- Eats few, if any, animal products (one or two servings per week at most) and chooses healthier options in this food group.

- Avoid foods that are completely empty of nutrients

or toxic for the body, such as sugar, sweeteners, white flour, processed foods and fast foods.

The Nutritarian way to health, longevity and weight loss focuses on the healthy foods with the strongest evidence supporting their anticancer and longevity-promoting effects. These are green vegetables, particularly leafy green cruciferous vegetables, along with beans, onions, mushrooms, berries, and seeds. These are the foods that have documented benefits to prevent cancer and other diseases. Remember this acronym:

G-BOMBS

Greens, Beans, Onions, Mushrooms, Berries and Seeds

A Nutritarian is someone who learns to trust the amazing power of the body. If given half a chance, the body will heal itself—with the right food as the catalyst. When you learn how to become a Nutritarian, you will arm yourself with the biochemical sustenance that your body needs to be at its ideal weight and to live a healthy, empowered life.

Finally, a Nutritarian lifestyle is an attitude, a mindset, a method that can be followed for a lifetime. As you begin your journey as a Nutritarian, you will be empowered to take control of your own health and life.

Vegetarian, Flexitarian or Nutritarian

The foundation of the Nutritarian diet is vegetables and other high-nutrient foods, but it does not have to be at the exclusion of all animal foods. A vegan diet is one that contains no foods of animal product origin, whereas a vegetarian diet may contain some dairy and eggs. A vegetarian or vegan diet can be an option for excellent health, as long as care is taken to eat healthful, nutrient-rich foods. However, a vegetarian or vegan who lives on processed cereals, white flour products, white rice, white potato and processed soy products is still vulnerable to the weight gain, diseases and many of the other complications resulting from the standard American diet because their diet cannot be considered nutrient-rich.

Being a Nutritarian differs from being a typical vegan because the focus isn't on totally excluding animal foods. The focus is on including the high-nutrient foods a body needs to improve health dramatically. A Nutritarian can reduce the level of animal products to a safe level without having to exclude them completely. A Nutritarian could be a vegan or not. Eating this way makes either option healthful.

The Nutritarian Difference

The Nutritarian diet is different because it doesn't require deprivation, starvation or denying your body foods that properly nourish it. It truly is a whole new way of looking at food. This handbook will show you why nutrient-rich foods are so powerful and will help you learn exactly what to eat and how to incorporate these foods into your diet.

Your body can change in amazing and dramatic ways. Many people who have adopted the Nutritarian lifestyle have reversed diet-related diseases such as diabetes, heart disease, chronic fatigue, autoimmune disease and migraines. The right food can be the most healing "medicine" you put in your body.

Whether you want to lose weight or just eat more healthfully, an easy way to make the right dietary choices is to sort foods into three categories:

Eat Liberally

Eat in Moderation

Avoid Entirely

Note that the term "eat liberally" is more accurate than the term "unlimited." Unlimited could imply overeating, or recreational or emotional eating, or eating when not hungry. Also, consuming too much of a very healthy food, such as fruit, can lead to insufficient vegetables in your diet.

The Nutritarian diet encourages liberal consumption of raw vegetables, cooked green and non-green, nutrient-dense vegetables, fruit, and beans. Raw nuts and seeds are included in the diet, but in limited quantities if weight loss is a goal. Starchy vegetables and whole grains are also included in the diet, but in limited amounts.

Products made with refined sugar and refined white fiber are off-limits, as well as barbecued, processed and cured meat, and all red meat and cheese. These foods provide few antioxidants and phytochemicals, and decrease the nutrient density of your diet. Significant quantities of high-protein foods also drive up hormones linked to higher rates of breast, prostate and colon cancer.

Foods to Eat Liberally, Eat in Moderation or Avoid Entirely
Eat Liberally
You can eat as much as you want of these foods (within reason):
- **Raw vegetables** (*Goal: about 1 pound daily*)
- **Cooked green and non-green nutrient dense vegetables** (*Goal: about ½ to 1 pound daily*) Non-green nutrient dense veggies are: tomatoes, cauliflower, eggplant, mushrooms, peppers, onions and carrots
- **Beans, legumes, lentils, tempeh, edamame** (*Goal: ½-1 cup daily*)
- **Fresh or frozen fruit** (*3 to 5 servings per day; 1 serving should be berries. One serving = 1 piece or 1 ½ cups berries or chopped fruit.*)

Limited (Eat in Moderation)
Include these foods in your diet but limit the amount you are eating.
- **Cooked starchy vegetables or whole grains** (*Maximum: 2 servings daily; 1 serving = 1 cup or 1*

slice; limit bread items to no more than 3 servings per week)

- Butternut and other winter squashes
- Potatoes, corn or wild rice
- Quinoa other intact whole grains
- 100% whole grain bread

•**Raw nuts and seeds** Half should be walnuts or chia, hemp, flax or sesame seeds (Eat at least 1 ounce or ¼ cup per day; if trying to lose weight, limit to a maximum of 1.5 ounces for women and 2 ounces for men per day)

- Avocado (Maximum ½ per day)
- Tofu (½-1 cup daily))
- Dried Fruit (Maximum 2 tablespoons per day)
- Animal Products: fat-free dairy, wild fish and certified organic poultry (Maximum of 6 ounces per week, limit each serving size to 2 ounces and use as a minor component/flavoring agent). Eggs (not more than two eggs per week)

Note: If you are not trying to lose weight, amounts of cooked starchy vegetables, intact whole grains, nuts, seeds and avocado may be increased depending on your caloric needs.

Off-Limits

- **Products made with refined sugar and refined white flour**
- **Soda and soft drinks** including those made with artificial sweeteners

- **Fruit Juice** (except pomegranate juice)
- **Barbecued, processed and cured meats and all red meat**
- **Full-fat and reduced-fat dairy** (cheese, ice cream, butter, milk)
- **Oils such as olive oil and other vegetable oil**

Note: *If you are not trying to lose weight, a small amount of olive oil may be used – but aim for a maximum of 1 table-spoon/week. See recommendations on Page 45.*

CHAPTER THREE

THE HEALTH EQUATION

Discovering Nutrients

There are two kinds of nutrients: macronutrients and micronutrients. Macronutrients are protein, carbohydrate, fat (and water). Excluding water, they are the three calorie-containing nutrients. The right food is your best medicine.

Micronutrients are vitamins, minerals and phytochemicals and are calorie-free. Obviously, we need to consume both kinds of nutrients, but the American diet contains too many macronutrients and not enough micronutrients.

MACRONUTRIENTS = FAT, CARBOHYDRATE & PROTEIN
CONTAIN CALORIES
SHOULD LIMIT CONSUMPTION

MICRONUTRIENTS = VITAMINS, MINERALS & PHYTOCHEMICALS
DO NOT CONTAIN CALORIES
SHOULD INCREASE CONSUMPTION

Eating foods that are naturally rich in micronutrients is the secret to achieving optimal health and super immunity. A micronutrient-heavy diet supplies your body with 14 different vitamins, 25 different minerals, and more than 10,000 phytochemicals, which are plant-based chemicals that have profound effects on human cell function and the immune system. Foods that are naturally rich in these nutrients are also rich in fiber and water, and are naturally low in calories, meaning they have a low caloric density. These low-calorie, high-nutrient foods provide the ingredients that activate your body's self-healing and self-repairing mechanisms. They are nature's contribution to your health turnaround! The foundational principle of this program is that the right food is your best medicine.

About 80 years ago, when scientists first identified vitamins and minerals, they thought they could have a profound effect on reducing risks of cancer and other life-shortening diseases. Businesses started to pop up touting the health benefits of different isolated vitamins and minerals. When the fortification of foods and the explosion of the supplement industry became a major contributor to America's micronutrient pie, an amazing thing happened: Cancer rates increased for 70 years straight, from 1935 to 2005.[10] Cancer incidence and mortality rates are continuing to climb worldwide. Isolating vitamins and minerals is not the answer.

Later, scientists discovered phytonutrients. Shockingly, natural foods contained many more critical nutritional elements than was ever imagined. With thousands of nutrients in a strawberry or piece of broccoli, nutrient intake is more intricate than originally thought. When the right assortment of natural foods is consumed, these nutrients work harmoniously to increase our immunity and protect our body against disease.

The phytochemical revolution

All the different types of nutrients are vital to achieving and maintaining optimal health and nutritional excellence; however, phytochemicals hold a special, elite place in the nutritional landscape. When consistently consumed in adequate quantity and variety, phytochemicals become super-nutrients in your body. They work together to detoxify cancer-causing compounds, deactivate free radicals, protect against radiation damage and enable DNA repair mechanisms.[11] When altered or broken strands of DNA are repaired, it can prevent cancer from developing later in life.

Consuming phytochemicals is not optional. They are essential in human immune-system defenses. Without a wide variety and sufficient amount of phytochemicals from unprocessed plant foods, scientists note that cells age more rapidly and do not retain their innate ability to remove and detoxify waste products and toxic compounds.

Low levels of phytochemical-rich produce in our modern diet are largely responsible for the common diseases seen with aging. We have learned so much from modern nutritional science in recent years, and when applied to our daily life, it works: We can live longer and better, with almost no risk of the diseases that plague most Americans.

Let's take heart disease as an example. Heart attacks are extremely rare occurrences in populations that eat a diet rich in protective phytochemicals (from vegetables) such as the Okinawans of Japan, but are omnipresent in populations, such as ours, that eat a diet low in these protective nutrients. Compelling data from numerous population studies shows that a natural, plant-based diet rich in antioxidants and phytochemicals will prevent, arrest, and even reverse heart disease.[12]

Our bodies were designed to make use of thousands of plant compounds. When these necessary compounds are missing, we survive because our bodies are adaptable; but over time, we lose our powerful potential for wellness, and chronic disease develops. We are robbed of living to our fullest potential in good physical, emotional, and mental health. Consumption of healthy foods leads to disease resistance; consumption of unhealthy foods makes us disease-prone.

Eating right enables you to feel your best every day. You may still get sick from a virus, but your body will be in a far better position to defend itself and make a quick and complete recovery. Optimal nutrition enables us to work better, play better, and maintain our youthful vigor as we age gracefully.

The Health Equation

The secret to a long life and disease reversal is to eat a diet lower in calories but higher in nutrients. It is all about nutrient bang per caloric buck. This important nutritional concept can be presented by a simple mathematical formula, which I call my health equation.

DR. FUHRMAN'S HEALTH EQUATION:
$$H = N/C$$

Your **Health** is dependent on the **Nutrient-per-Calorie** density of your diet.

In this discussion, the word "nutrient" refers to micronutrients. Your future health equals nutrient consumption divided by calories. This straightforward mathematical formula is the basis of nutritional science and nutritional healing. This formula essentially states that for you to be in excellent health, your diet must be nutrient-rich, and you must not overeat on calories (or macronutrients). The nutrient density in your body's tissues is proportional to the nutrient density of your diet. We realize we must seek out and consume more foods with a high nutrient-per-calorie density and fewer foods with a low nutrient-per-calorie density.[13]

Every nutritional scientist in the world agrees that moderate caloric restriction in the environment of micronutrient adequacy slows the aging process, prevents the development of chronic diseases, and extends lifespan. This has been tested in every species of animal, including primates.[14] There is no controversy that Americans are eating themselves to death with too many calories. To change this we must do three things:

1 - EAT LESS FAT
2 - EAT LESS PROTEIN
3 - EAT LESS CARBOHYDRATE

Even though reduction of calories is valuable, the focus here is different. When the fatty foods you eat are high-nutrient fatty foods, and the proteins you eat are high-nutrient proteins, and the carbohydrates you eat are high-nutrient carbohydrates, you naturally desire fewer calories. Natural, whole plant foods are a mixture of fat, carbohydrate and protein and in their natural state, they are typically rich in micronutrients. Simply trying to reduce calories is called dieting, and dieting doesn't work. The reason this program is so successful is because over time, without even trying or noticing it, you will prefer to eat fewer calories. I know that can sound unlikely. Many people think: "Not me" or "My body doesn't work that way" or "It will be a real struggle for me." However, if you follow the plan, it will happen instinctually and almost effortlessly. I have seen it happen to thousands, with all kinds of different backgrounds and eating histories. I promise, it can happen for you, too.

This program will help you achieve superior health and lose weight if you need to, by eating more nutrient-rich foods and fewer high-calorie, low-nutrient foods. **It works because the more high-nutrient food you consume, the less low-nutrient food you desire.** Foods are nutrient-dense when they contain a high level of micronutrients per calorie. Green vegetables win the award for the most nutrient-dense foods on the planet. Therefore, as you move forward in your quest for nutritional excellence, you will eat more and more vegetables. Since they contain the most nutrients per calorie, vegetables have the most powerful association with life extension and protection from heart disease and cancer.

It is also important to achieve micronutrient diversity. This means obtaining enough of all beneficial nutrients, not merely higher amounts of a select few. Eating a variety of plant foods is the key to achieving micronutrient diversity. Consider mushrooms and onions to illustrate this concept. They may not contain the highest amounts of vitamins and minerals, but they contain a significant amount of unique, protective phytochemicals that are not found in other foods.

Test Your Nutrient IQ

How smart are you when it comes to making nutrient-dense food choices? You can find out by using my new food-scoring system, called **Nutrient IQ**. Nutrient IQ is a scoring system that allows you to rate your diet by adding up points for the day. Foods are assigned points based on their nutrient content and contribution to good health. You can adjust the points based on the size of the serving you eat.

As you might expect, the foods that have a high Nutrient IQ score are straight from nature—primarily vegetables, fruit and legumes, while refined, processed foods provide few or no points. Even though attention should be placed on nutrient-rich foods, it is also important to achieve micronutrient diversity and to eat an adequate assortment of lower-ranked plant foods in order to obtain the full range of human dietary requirements. Try to include some Greens, Beans, Onions, Mushrooms, Berries and Seeds in your diet every day. Think G-BOMBS!

Because phytochemicals are largely unnamed and unmeasured, these rankings may underestimate the healthful properties of colorful, natural plant foods, so the comparative nutrient density of many of these whole foods may be even higher than these scores indicate.

The Nutrient IQ point system differs from the ANDI (Aggregate Nutrient Density Index) scores I have published in previous books. ANDI provides a ranking of foods based on the nutrients contained in an equal-calorie serving of each food. Foods are ranked on a scale of 1 to 1,000 with the most nutrient- dense leafy, cruciferous vegetables scoring at 1000. The Nutrient IQ score is different because it is connected to specific serving sizes of foods. This enables you to add up your scores and get a personal dietary rating each day.

Nutrient IQ encourages you to make better food choices and allows you to see how your diet varies from day to day. It demonstrates the nutritional value of colorful plants compared with that of animal products, oils, and processed foods. In case you haven't guessed, selecting a variety of vegetables, fruit and beans will provide the highest daily scores.

Use these target scores to see how your diet measures up:

DAILY TARGET SCORES

	Men	Women
Smart	600	500
Brilliant	800	650
Genius	1000	800

Improving your daily score is about making better, more nutrient-dense food choices, not eating more food.

To move up from Smart to Brilliant to Genius, you need to increase your servings of green leafy vegetables and cruciferous vegetables and make sure your daily menus include a well-rounded assortment of other high-nutrient IQ vegetables as well as beans, fruit, berries and seeds.

The serving sizes listed in the table below and in Chapter Six are convenient measurements; they are not necessarily recommended serving amounts. Adjust your scores based on the amount of the food that you eat. For example, the table lists 90 points for 1 cup of broccoli, so if you have 2 cups, give yourself 180 points. If a medium tomato is worth 60 points, then give yourself 30 points for eating half. If a vegetable, fruit, bean or whole grain food you are looking for is not listed in the table, assign it a value based on a similar food item. Assume that most processed, refined foods and anything made with refined white flour and white sugar provide zero points.

Please note that you do **NOT** have to score foods and keep track of points to eat a Nutritarian diet and be healthy. You do not have to keep track of your calories. This is a motivational tool to help you to learn how to eat more healthfully. You only have to understand how to lay out a healthful and nutritionally balanced menu, and then stick to it.

Matter of Emphasis

Most health authorities today are in agreement that we should add more servings of healthy fruits and vegetables to our diet. I disagree. Thinking about our diet in this fashion doesn't adequately address the problem. Instead of adding those protective fruits, vegetables, beans, seeds and nuts to our disease-causing diet, these foods must be the main focus of the diet itself. This is what makes the Nutritarian approach different.

Once we understand that concept, then we can add a few servings of foods that are not in this category to the diet each week, and use animal products as condiments or small additions to this naturally nutrient-rich diet. The following chart provides a sample of Nutrient IQ scores for several different foods. Please refer to Chapter Six for additional scores.

SAMPLE NUTRIENT IQ SCORES

Kale, cooked	1 cup	112
Broccoli	1 cup	90
Romaine	2 cups	64
Tomato	1 medium	60
Mushrooms	¼ cup	60
Onions, raw	¼ cup	60
Beans	½ cup	52
Carrots	1 cup	45
Corn	1 cup	45
Strawberries	½ cup	45
Flax seeds	1 tablespoon	41
Quinoa	1 cup	26
White Potato	1 medium	12
Salmon	4 ounces	7
Chicken breast	4 ounces	4
White Pasta		0
Olive Oil		0

Chapter Four

THREE LEVELS OF SUPERIOR NUTRITION

I have organized meal plans into three levels of superior nutrition. Based on your health needs and current dietary habits, you can choose between three different diet options.

Level One: Smart
Level Two: Brilliant
Level Three: Genius

I would like to see everyone reach at least Level Two, although for many, even Level One will represent a significant improvement. Use the Nutrient IQ scores contained in Chapter Six of this book to help you choose the most nutrient-dense foods. You will find sample menus and healthy recipes in Chapters Seven and Eight of this handbook. High-nutrient density soups, delicious vegetable smoothies and healthy dressings and dips are featured in all my meal plans, however this handbook only gives a sample of the valuable information. More menus and recipes are available in my books, including *Eat for Life*, *The Eat to Live Cookbook*, and the *Eat to Live Quick and Easy Cookbook*. You will also find meal plans and recipes on my website, www. DrFuhrman.com.

I have designed three levels, as an aid to direct people to the level of nutritional excellence they need for their individual health conditions. This does not mean a person should not move to a higher level of excellence if they are comfortable doing so.

Regardless of what level you choose, take a 28-day Nutritarian Pledge to follow these cornerstones of healthy eating:

Include daily:
1) A large salad
2) At least a half-cup serving of beans/legumes in soup, salad or a main dish
3) At least three fresh fruits
4) At least one ounce (total) of raw nuts and seeds
5) At least one large (double-size) serving of steamed green vegetables

Avoid:
1) Barbecued, processed and red meat
2) Fried foods
3) Dairy (cheese, ice cream, butter, whole milk and 2% milk)
4) Soft drinks, sugar and other sweetening agents or artificial sweeteners

5) White flour products
6) Oil

The point is to give your body a real chance to change its biochemistry and build up its nutrient stores. You will see how much better your life can be when you are well nourished.

Level 1: Smart (Men: 600 points, Women: 500 points)

Level 1 is appropriate for a person who is healthy, thin, physically fit and exercises regularly. You should have no risk factors such as high blood pressure, high cholesterol or a family history of heart disease, stroke or cancer before the age of 75. Most Americans do have risk factors or a family history of strokes, heart attacks and cancer, and most Americans are overweight. So most people should only see Level 1 as a temporary stage as they learn about high-nutrient eating and allow their taste buds to acclimate to higher levels of whole, natural plant foods.

Level 1 is designed to ease the emotional shock of making profound dietary improvements. It enables people to revamp their diet at a level that is significant, but not overwhelming. Enjoy this new style of eating, allow your taste preferences to change with time, and learn some great recipes. You may soon decide to move to a higher level. However, I still recommend that the majority of individuals make the commitment to jump right into the more nutrient-dense Levels 2 or 3 because so many people are significantly overweight and have risk factors that need to be addressed immediately. People in desperate need of a health makeover need to start on Levels 2 or 3.

On Level 1, you eliminate fried foods, and substitute fruit-based healthful desserts and whole grains for low-nutrient processed snack foods such as salty snacks, candy, ice cream and baked products. Whole grain products like old fashioned oats, quinoa and 100% whole grain bread are used. Bread products made with refined white flour are eliminated. Pasta made with white flour is replaced with bean pasta.

Your sodium intake will decrease as you begin to make these dietary changes. Processed foods and restaurant foods contribute 77 percent of the sodium people consume. Salt from the saltshaker provides 11 percent and sodium found naturally in food provides the remaining 12 percent.[15]

You also eliminate foods like cheese and butter that are high in saturated fats. Your cooking techniques use only a minimal amount of oil. Most Americans consume over 20 servings of animal products weekly. In Level 1, I recommend only four servings of animal products per week. These animal products are limited to fish, skinless chicken or turkey, eggs or nonfat dairy products.

Level 2: Brilliant (Men: 800 points, Women: 650 points)
Level 2 builds on the positive changes described in Level 1. In Level 2, animal products are reduced to three servings weekly and vegetables and beans should start to make up an even larger portion of your total caloric intake. When you incorporate more and more nutrient-rich produce in your diet, you automatically increase your intake of antioxidants, phytochemicals, plant fibers, and plant sterols. You lower the glycemic index of your diet and the level of saturated fat, salt and other negative elements without having to think about it. Your ability to appreciate the

natural flavors of unprocessed, whole foods will improve with time because you lose your dependence on salt and sugar. Add more beans and nuts to your diet to replace animal products.

Try some of the high-nutrient dressing and dip recipes in Chapter Eight. They use heart-healthy nuts and seeds to replace the oils found in traditional dressings and dips.

Level 2 is a reasonable target diet for most people. If you want to lose weight, lower your cholesterol, lower your blood pressure or just live a long and healthy life, this is the level you should adopt.

How much you should eat varies widely from person to person, but if you are not at your ideal weight, you should be moving closer to achieving it every day. If you are significantly overweight or obese, you should be losing at least two pounds a week on your way to recovery. You will find that the better you adhere to a nutrient-dense, plant-rich diet style, the more your hunger sensations are transformed and you simply desire fewer calories.

Level 3: Genius (Men: 1000 points, Women: 800 points)

If you suffer from serious medical conditions such as diabetes, heart disease, or autoimmune disease, or just want to optimize the nutrient density of your diet to slow aging and maximize longevity, step up to Level 3. If you suffer from a medical condition that is important to reverse, this is the right prescription for you. If you are on medications and you want to be able to discontinue them as quickly as possible, go for Level 3. It is also the level to choose if you have trouble losing weight, no matter what you do, and want to maximize your results.

Level 3 is designed for those who want to reverse serious disease, or for healthy people who want to push the envelope of human longevity. Level 3 is the diet that I use in my medical practice for people who have serious autoimmune diseases; (such as rheumatoid arthritis or lupus), or when someone has life-threatening heart disease (atherosclerosis). I prescribe it for diabetics who need to lower their blood sugars into the normal range, or to get rid of severe migraines. It delivers the highest level of nutrient density.

Level 3 includes a maximum of two small servings of animal products weekly and concentrates on vegetables with high nutrient density. Use the Nutrient IQ scores in Chapter Six to select the most nutrient-dense foods possible. Use green smoothies, fresh vegetable juices, healthful soups and lots of greens and raw vegetables to make every calorie count.

At this level, you should consume processed foods only rarely. Keep the use of refined fats and oils to a minimum. Nuts and seeds supply essential fats in a much healthier package, with significant health benefits. The menus and recipes in Chapters Seven and Eight provide some ideas for incorporating a variety of nutrient dense foods into your diet.

In the following table, I have listed some of the top foods in the six food categories that should make up 75-80 percent of your diet. These foods get some of the highest Nutrient IQ scores. Below each group, the number of servings suggested to achieve Level 1, 2 or 3 is listed. These amounts should not be seen as rigid requirements, but rather as helpful guidelines. Of course there are many other choices in these categories and I encourage you to try them all.

Three Levels of Superior Nutrition

Recommended Servings of Vegetables, Fruit, Beans and Nuts

COOKED GREEN VEGETABLES

1.5 cups kale

1.5 cups mustard, turnip or collard greens

1.5 cups bok choy

1.5 cups broccoli rabe

1.5 cups spinach

1.5 cups Brussels sprouts

1.5 cups Swiss chard

1.5 cups broccoli

1.5 cups cabbage

LEVEL ONE	LEVEL TWO	LEVEL THREE
1-2 servings	2-3 servings	2-3 servings

RAW GREEN VEGETABLES

3 cups watercress

5 cups spinach

5 cups romaine, Boston, red or green leaf lettuce

5 cups arugula

5 cups mixed baby greens

1.5 cups raw broccoli

1.5 cups cabbage

1.5 cups green pepper

2 cups zucchini

1.5 cups snow peas

LEVEL ONE	LEVEL TWO	LEVEL THREE
1 serving	1-2 servings	2-3 servings

NON-GREEN VEGETABLES

1 cup carrots	1 tomato
6 radishes	1/2 cup chopped onion or scallions
1 cup red pepper	
2 cups radicchio	1/2 cup cooked mushrooms
1 cup cauliflower	

LEVEL ONE	LEVEL TWO	LEVEL THREE
1 serving	1-2 servings	1-2 servings

FRUIT

1.5 cups strawberries	1.5 cups cantaloupe
1.5 cups raspberries	2 kiwis
1.5 cups blueberries	2.5 cups watermelon
2 plums	1 apple
1 orange	1.5 cups cherries

LEVEL ONE	LEVEL TWO	LEVEL THREE
3-5 servings	3-5 servings	3-5 servings

BEANS

1/2 - 1 cup lentils

1/2 - 1 cup red kidney

1/2 - 1 cup black beans

1/2 - 1 cup pinto beans

1/2 - 1 cup split peas

1/2 - 1 cup edamame

1/2 - 1 cup chickpeas

1/2 - 1 cup white beans

1 cup cooked bean pasta

4 oz tempeh

LEVEL ONE	LEVEL TWO	LEVEL THREE
1-3 servings	1-3 servings	1-3 servings

NUTS AND SEEDS

1/4 cup sunflower seeds

2 tablespoons ground flax, hemp or chia seeds

1/4 cup sesame seeds

1/4 cup pumpkin seeds

1/4 cup pistachios

1/4 cup pecans

1/4 cup almonds

1/4 cup walnuts

1/4 cup cashews

2 tablespoons raw nut or seed butter

LEVEL ONE	LEVEL TWO	LEVEL THREE
1-3 servings*	1-3 servings*	1-3 servings*

* The amount of nuts and seeds as well as other foods you consume depends on your caloric requirements. If you are trying to lose weight, limit nuts to one serving daily. If you are thin, want to gain weight or need more calories to fuel your athletic activities, then the number of servings may be increased.

Eating enough healthy food is critical to your success as a Nutritarian. You will find that when you eat enough high-nutrient food, you no longer desire or even have room for the other foods that used to make up the biggest part of your diet. Processed and refined foods offer little in terms of nutrients and phytochemicals. When you eat them, you are missing the opportunity to eat other foods that contain valuable nutrients that could be put to good use by your body.

Overview of the Three Levels
Recommended Amounts

	LEVEL 1	LEVEL 2	LEVEL 3
VEGETABLES raw & cooked 1 serving = 1-1/2 cups cooked or 2 to 5 cups raw	3-4 servings/day	4-6 servings/day	5-7 servings/day
FRUIT 1 serving = about 1-1/2 cups	3-5 servings/day	3-5 servings/day	3-5 servings/day
BEANS 1 serving = 1/2 to 1 cup	1-2 servings/day	1-2 servings/day	1-2 servings/day
NUTS & SEEDS 1 serving = 1 ounce or 1/4 cup	1-3 servings/day	1-3 servings/day ————1 serving/day if trying to lose weight————	1-3 servings/day
WHOLE GRAIN PRODUCTS/POTATOES 1 serving = 1 slice or 1 cup	1-3 servings/day	1-2 servings/day	1-2 servings/day
ANIMAL PRODUCTS* 1 serving = 2 ounces	4 servings/week or less	3 servings/week or less	2 servings/week or less
SODIUM	1200 mg/day or less	1200 mg/day or less	1000 mg/day or less
FATS/OILS Avoid processed, refined fats and oil. A small amount of olive oil may be used if you are not trying to lose weight.	Maximum of 1 tablespoon of olive oil/day	Maximum of 2 tablespoons of olive oil/week	Maximum of 1 tablespoon of olive oil/week

* Animal products can be fat-free dairy, certified organic poultry or fish. Choose wild fish and lower mercury species such as salmon, sole, cod, trout, sardines, scallops, shrimp or lobster. Avoid red meat, and barbecued, processed and cured meats.

CHAPTER FIVE

TOP NUTRITARIAN PRINCIPLES

Here is my Top Ten list of Nutritarian principles.

1. Your body's immune system needs the right foods to allow it to work to its fullest potential.
By changing our diets and combining foods that contain powerful immune-strengthening capabilities, we can achieve incredible health and prevent and even reverse disease. The Standard American Diet is nutrient-deficient. We are eating too many highly processed foods, foods with added sweeteners and animal fats and proteins. At the same time, we are not eating enough fruits, vegetables, seeds and beans, which leaves us lacking in hundreds of the most immune-building compounds.

2. H=N/C — Dr. Fuhrman's Health Equation
Your long-term Health is directly related to the amount

of Nutrients you get for each Calorie you consume. The more "nutrient-dense" a food, the more powerful it is. The most nutrient-dense foods are fruits and vegetables, especially dark leafy greens which are the foods missing in most modern diets. Nutrient-dense foods contain vital nutrients, vitamins and minerals essential for preventing disease, boosting immunity, detoxifying the body and delivering permanent weight loss.

3. Prescription medications will not solve your health problems.

Heart disease, Type II diabetes, hypertension and many other conditions are directly related to poor dietary habits. The body has an incredible ability to heal itself when properly nourished. For example, even patients on insulin for years can reduce and eventually eliminate medications as they lose weight and become healthy. Superior nutrition is more effective than medications at resolving most medical problems while promoting a pleasurable, longer and more healthful life.

4. If you want to lose weight — DON'T DIET!

Ninety-five percent of all weight lost on most popular diets is regained. While many diets may produce short-term weight loss, they cannot be maintained and therefore the weight returns. The only proven strategy for permanent weight loss is to consume sufficient nutrients and fiber for a lifetime of excellent health. This strategy will reduce your cravings for "junk'" food and curb the tendency to overeat. You will instinctually eat fewer calories, without the food addictions and cravings that have sabotaged your attempts in the past.

5. Where's the Beef?
Remember that vegetables, beans and seeds are high in protein, so there is no essential need to have animal products for protein. Think about it: Cows are vegan, as are gorillas and horses. Trying to lose weight or reduce your cholesterol? Think greens for health and for building lean muscle. To maximize our health and longevity, we need to get more protein from nutrient-rich plant sources such as greens, beans, seeds and nuts and less from animal products.

6. Remember: G-BOMBS
Greens, Beans, Onions, Mushrooms, Berries and Seeds are important foods with powerful immune-strengthening capabilities. Include these super foods in your diet every day.

7. Watch the Olive Oil!
One tablespoon of olive oil has 120 calories (all oils do). One-quarter cup has 500 calories. Healthy salads are definitely a way of life for people who want to lose weight or

improve health. However, many of the benefits of a salad are lost when the calorie count is increased ten-fold with refined oil. Nut and seed-based dressings are the way to go. Nuts and seeds, not oil, have shown dramatic protection against heart disease. We need to get more of our fats from these wholesome foods and less from processed oils.

8. If health came in a bottle, we'd all be healthy!

Natural, whole, plant-based foods are highly complex. It may never be possible to extract the precise symphony of nutrients found in fruits and vegetables and place it in a pill. So don't rely on pills and supplements to get your primary nutrition.

9. Six-A-Day – Not the Way!

You have probably heard it's better to eat six small meals a day. That is not ideal. You simply will not need to eat that frequently once your body is well nourished with micronutrients. The body can more effectively detoxify and enhance cell repair when not constantly eating and digesting. Eating healthfully removes cravings and reduces the sensations driving us to eat too much and too often. For most people who follow a Nutritarian diet-style, eating when truly hungry means eating three or maybe two meals a day.

10. Let Your Body Decide!

Nobody wants to hear that they have to give up all their favorite foods, such as pizza and ice cream. But wouldn't it be nice if over time your body actually preferred healthy foods? The body can change its taste and food preferences. As you consume larger and larger portions of health-promoting foods, your appetite for low-nutrient foods decreases and you gradually lose your addiction to sugar and fats. You learn to enjoy and prepare gourmet-tasting meals that are nutrient-rich. When this occurs, you have become a Nutritarian!

I realize unhealthy foods can be very appealing and hard to resist. Please be patient with yourself as you start to eat right. As you switch to healthful foods, you will lose your cravings for unhealthful foods. You will learn to eat only when you are truly hungry. Your body will learn to love fresh fruits and vegetables and my healthful recipes because they taste so great and are satisfying.

Becoming a Nutritarian is all about having the knowledge and support you need to get back in touch with the natural wisdom of your body.

CHAPTER SIX

NUTRIENT IQ SCORES

	CALORIES	SODIUM	NUT. IQ
VEGETABLES			
Kale, cooked (1 cup)	43	19	112
Mustard Greens, cooked (1 cup)	36	13	112
Collard Greens, cooked (1 cup)	63	29	112
Turnip Greens, cooked (1 cup)	29	42	112
Swiss Chard, cooked (1 cup)	35	313	112
Watercress, cooked (1 cup)	15	373	112
Broccoli, raw (1 cup)	31	30	90
Broccoli, cooked (1 cup)	55	64	90
Broccoli rabe, raw (1 cup)	9	13	90
Broccoli rabe, cooked (1 cup)	43	95	90
Bok choy, raw (1 cup)	9	46	90

	CALORIES	SODIUM	NUT. IQ
Bok choy, cooked (1 cup)	20	58	90
Brussels sprouts, raw (1 cup)	38	22	90
Brussels sprouts, cooked (1 cup)	56	33	90
Cauliflower, raw (1 cup)	27	32	90
Cauliflower, cooked (1 cup)	29	32	90
Cabbage, cooked (1 cup)			
(green, red, napa, savoy)	34	12	90
Kohlrabi, raw (1 cup)	36	27	90
Kohlrabi, cooked (1 cup)	48	35	90
Radishes, raw (1 cup)	19	45	90
Turnips, raw (1 cup)	36	87	90
Turnips, cooked (1 cup)	34	25	90
Spinach, cooked (1 cup)	41	126	82
Endive, cooked (1 cup)	23	29	82
Escarole, cooked (1 cup)	23	29	82
Kale, raw (1 cup)	7	11	79
Mustard greens, raw (1 cup)	15	11	79
Collard greens, raw (1 cup)	12	6	79
Turnip greens, raw (1 cup)	18	22	79
Swiss chard, raw (1 cup)	7	77	79
Watercress, raw (1 cup)	4	14	79
Arugula, raw (1 cup)	5	5	79
Cabbage, raw, 1 cup			
(green, red, napa, savoy)	22	16	79

	CALORIES	SODIUM	NUT. IQ
Spinach, raw (2 cups)	14	47	64
Endive, raw (2 cups)	9	11	64
Escarole, raw (2 cups)	13	18	64
Romaine lettuce (2 cups)	13	18	64
Red or green leaf lettuce (2 cups)	14	14	64
Boston or Bibb lettuce (2 cups)	7	3	64
Mixed baby greens (2 cups)	12	20	64
Asparagus, raw (1 cup)	27	3	64
Asparagus, cooked (1 cup)	40	25	64
Artichokes (1 item)	64	120	64
Artichokes (3/4 cup hearts)	67	108	64
Cucumber (1 cup)	17	3	64
Fennel, raw (1 cup)	27	45	64
Green beans, raw (1 cup)	31	6	64
Green beans, cooked (1 cup)	44	1	64
Green pepper, raw (1 cup)	18	3	64
Green pepper, cooked (1 cup)	38	3	64
Okra, cooked (1 cup)	35	10	64
Snow peas, raw (1 cup)	27	3	64
Snow peas, cooked (1 cup)	67	6	64
Sugar snap peas, raw (1 cup)	27	3	64
Sugar snap peas, cooked (1 cup)	67	6	64
Zucchini, raw (1 cup)	21	10	64
Zucchini, cooked (1 cup)	27	5	64

	CALORIES	SODIUM	NUT. IQ
Bean sprouts, raw (1 cup)	31	6	60
Bean sprouts, cooked (1 cup)	62	11	60
Eggplant, cooked (1 cup)	35	1	60
Red pepper, raw (1 cup)	39	6	60
Red Pepper, cooked (1 cup)	38	1	60
Tomatoes, raw (1 cup or 1 medium tomato)	32	9	60
Tomatoes, cooked (1 cup)	43	26	60
Tomato sauce, no-salt-added (1 cup)	78	37	60
Pasta sauce, low-sodium (1 cup)	131	77	60
Tomato paste (1 tablespoon)	13	9	6
Radicchio, raw (1 cup)	9	9	60
Yellow squash, raw (1 cup)	18	2	60
Yellow squash, cooked (1 cup)	36	2	60
Mushrooms, cooked (1/4 cup)	11	1	60
Onions, raw (1/4 cup)	16	2	60
Shallots, raw (1/4 cup)	29	1	60
Scallions/green onions, raw (1/4 cup)	8	4	60
Leeks, raw (1/4 cup)	14	5	60
Garlic, raw (1/4 cup)	51	6	60
Garlic, raw (1 clove)	5	1	5
Beets, raw (1 cup)	59	106	45
Beets, cooked (1 cup)	75	65	45
Corn, cooked (1 cup)	143	1	45
Carrots, raw (1 cup)	53	88	45

	CALORIES	SODIUM	NUT. IQ
Carrots, raw (1 medium)	25	42	23
Carrots, cooked (1 cup)	55	45	45
Green peas, cooked (1 cup)	134	5	45
Pumpkin, cooked (1 cup)	49	2	45
Parsnips, cooked (1 cup)	55	8	45
Rutabaga, cooked (1 cup)	51	9	45
Potato, sweet, cooked (1 cup or 1 medium)	180	72	45
Butternut squash, cooked (1 cup)	82	8	45
Acorn squash, cooked (1 cup)	115	8	45
Spaghetti squash, cooked (1 cup)	42	28	45
Onions, shallots and green onions, cooked (1/4 cup)	23	6	30
Leeks, cooked (1/4 cup)	8	3	30
Garlic, cooked (1/4 cup)	49	21	30
Salsa, no-salt-added (1/4 cup)	19	4	26
Turmeric, ground (1 teaspoon)	9	1	25
Turmeric, fresh, chopped (1 tablespoon)	24	0	25
Avocado (1/4 cup or 1/4 avocado)	60	3	23
Potato, white, cooked (1 cup or 1 medium)	113	6	12
Celery, raw (1/2 cup)	7	81	11
Celery, cooked (1/2 cup)	27	136	11
Iceberg lettuce (2 cups)	16	11	11
Basil, fresh, chopped (2 tablespoons)	1	0	10
Dill, fresh, chopped (2 tablespoons)	1	0	10
Parsley, fresh, chopped (2 tablespoons)	3	4	10

	CALORIES	SODIUM	NUT. IQ
Cilantro, fresh, chopped (2 tablespoons)	1	1	10
Ginger root, fresh, chopped (1 tablespoon)	10	1	10
Cinnamon, ground (1 teaspoon)	6	0	10

FRUIT

	CALORIES	SODIUM	NUT. IQ
Strawberries (1/2 cup)	27	2	45
Blueberries (1/2 cup)	42	1	45
Raspberries (1/2 cup)	32	1	45
Blackberries (1/2 cup)	31	1	45
Cranberries, fresh not dried (1/2 cup)	23	1	45
Gooseberries (1/2 cup)	33	1	45
Goji berries, dried (1/2 cup)	156	133	45
Cherries, fresh (2/3 cup)	43	0	41
Pomegranate kernels (1/4 cup)	36	1	37
Pomegranate juice (1/4 cup)	34	6	37
Oranges (3/4 cup peeled sections or 1 medium)	62	0	19
Tangerines (3/4 cup peeled sections or 2 items)	77	3	19
Mandarin oranges (3/4 cup peeled sections or 2 items)	77	3	19
Clementines (3/4 cup peeled sections or 2 items)	70	1	19
Kumquats (4 items)	54	8	19
Grapefruit (1 cup or ½ grapefruit)	76	0	19
Watermelon (1 cup)	46	2	19
Cantaloupe (1 cup)	54	26	19

	CALORIES	SODIUM	NUT. IQ
Honeydew (1 cup)	61	31	19
Grapes (1 cup)	104	3	19
Papaya (1 cup)	62	12	19
Figs, fresh (2 figs)	74	1	19
Peaches (1 cup or 1 item)	60	0	19
Nectarines (1 cup or 1 item)	63	0	19
Apricots (1 cup or 2 items)	34	0	19
Plums (1 cup or 2 items)	61	0	19
Pears (1 cup or 1 item)	101	2	19
Mango (1 cup or ½ mango)	99	2	19
Pineapple (1 cup)	83	2	19
Kiwi (1 cup or 2 items)	84	4	19
Coconut, fresh (1 cup)	283	16	19
Apple (1 cup or 1 item)	95	2	11
Banana (1 cup or 1 item)	105	1	11

	CALORIES	SODIUM	NUT. IQ
DRIED FRUIT			
Blueberries, dried, unsweetened (1/4 cup)	129	0	8
Cherries, dried, unsweetened (1/4 cup)	118	24	8
Dates, (1/4 cup)	104	1	5
Dates (1 medjool date)	67	0	3
Dates (1 deglet noor date)	20	0	1
Raisins (1/4 cup)	109	4	5
Currants (1/4 cup)	102	3	5
Figs (1/4 cup)	93	4	5
Figs (1 fig)	21	1	2
Apricots (1/4 cup)	78	3	5
Coconut, dried, unsweetened (1/4 cup)	139	8	5
Cranberries, dried, sweetened (1/4 cup)	85	1	0
BEANS/LEGUMES			
Black, cooked (1/2 cup)	114	1	52
Cannellini, cooked (1/2 cup)	113	1	52
Chickpeas, cooked (1/2 cup)	135	6	52
Kidney, cooked (1/2 cup)	113	1	52
Navy, cooked (1/2 cup)	128	0	52
Lentils, cooked (1/2 cup)	115	2	52
Split peas, cooked (1/2 cup)	116	2	52
Edamame (1/2 cup)	65	3	52
Lima beans (1/2 cup)	108	2	52
Bean pasta, cooked (1 cup)	200	0	52
Bean pasta, dry (2 ounces)	200	0	52

	CALORIES	SODIUM	NUT. IQ
Tempeh (1 cup)	319	15	45
Hummus (1/4 cup)	146	149	35
Tofu (1 cup)	362	35	15
Soy milk (1 cup)	105	115	15

NUTS AND SEEDS

	CALORIES	SODIUM	NUT. IQ
Walnuts (1/4 cup)	164	0	45
Flax seeds (2 tablespoons)	112	6	41
Chia seeds (2 tablespoons)	99	3	41
Hemp seeds (2 tablespoons)	111	1	41
Pumpkin seeds (1/4 cup)	180	2	34
Sunflower seeds (1/4 cup)	204	3	34
Sesame seeds (1/4 cup)	206	4	34
Almonds (1/4 cup)	206	0	26
Brazil nuts (1/4 cup)	219	1	26
Cashews (1/4 cup)	188	4	26
Hazelnuts (1/4 cup)	212	0	26
Pecans (1/4 cup)	171	0	26
Pistachio nuts (1/4 cup)	172	0	26
Pine nuts (1/4 cup)	227	1	26
Macadamia nuts (1/4 cup)	240	2	15
Almond milk, unsweetened (1 cup)	37	173	15
Hemp milk, unsweetened (1 cup)	60	110	15
Coconut milk, unsweetened (1 cup)	45	70	15
Cashew butter (1 tablespoon)	94	2	13
Almond butter (1 tablespoon)	98	1	13

	CALORIES	SODIUM	NUT. IQ
Sunflower butter (1 tablespoon)	99	0	13
Tahini (1 tablespoon)	89	5	13
Peanuts, unsalted (1/4 cup)	219	2	11
Peanut butter, low sodium (1 tablespoon)	96	3	6

GRAINS

Whole Grains

Wild rice, cooked (1 cup)	101	3	26
Wild rice, dry (1/4 cup)	143	3	26
Steel cut oats, cooked (1 cup)	166	0	26
Steel cut oats, dry (1/4 cup)	150	0	26
Quinoa, cooked (1 cup)	222	13	26
Quinoa, dry (1/3 cup)	209	2	26
Buckwheat, cooked (1 cup)	155	7	26
Buckwheat, dry (1/4 cup)	146	2	26
Barley, cooked (1 cup)	198	5	26
Barley, dry (1/3 cup)	217	7	26
Bulgar, cooked (1 cup)	151	9	26
Teff, cooked (1 cup)	255	20	26
Farro, cooked (1 cup)	200	0	26
Farro, dry (1/3 cup)	211	0	26
Old fashioned oats, cooked (1 cup)	166	0	19
Old fashioned oats, dry (1/2 cup)	150	0	19
Cornmeal, dry(1/4 cup)	111	43	11

	CALORIES	SODIUM	NUT. IQ
Brown rice, cooked (1 cup)	248	8	7
Brown rice, uncooked (1/4 cup)	170	2	7
Bread, 100% whole grain (1 slice)	80	80	7
Pita, 100% whole grain (1 item)	90	110	7
Wraps, 100% whole grain (1 item)	150	140	7

REFINED GRAIN PRODUCTS

	CALORIES	SODIUM	NUT. IQ
Cold cereals (1 cup) made from 100% whole grains and nuts without added sweeteners	varies	varies	11
Cold cereals, not 100% whole grain	varies	varies	0
Pasta, whole wheat, cooked (1 cup)	186	7	7
Pasta, white, cooked	190	1	0
Couscous, cooked	176	8	0
Quick oats, cooked (1 cup)	166	9	4
Instant oats, cooked (1 cup)	230	266	4
Whole wheat bread products, not 100% whole wheat bread, wraps, pita, bagels	varies	varies	0
White bread products, all refined white flour bread, wraps, pita, bagels	varies	varies	0
Crackers	varies	varies	0

	CALORIES	SODIUM	NUT. IQ

DAIRY PRODUCTS AND EGGS

Eggs (1 item)	72	71	4
Milk, skim (1 cup)	83	102	4
Milk, 1% (1 cup)	102	107	4
Milk, 2% (1 cup)	122	115	3
Milk, whole (1 cup)	149	105	3
Plain Yogurt, fat free and low fat, no added sugar (6 ounces)	varies	varies	4
Plain Yogurt, full fat, no added sugar (6 ounces)	varies	varies	3
Yogurt with added sugar	varies	varies	0
Frozen yogurt	varies	varies	0
Cheese, all varieties (2 ounces)	varies	varies	2
Ice cream	varies	varies	0

FISH AND MEAT

Wild salmon (4 ounces)	207	63	7
Farmed salmon (4 ounces)	233	69	5
Lower mercury shellfish (4 ounces) scallops, clams, mussels, oysters, shrimp, lobster, crawfish	varies	varies	5
Lower mercury fish (4 ounces) sole, flounder, cod, bass, haddock, hake, sardine, trout,			

	CALORIES	SODIUM	NUT. IQ
squid, catfish, tilapia, mackerel, squid	varies	varies	5
All other seafood (4 ounces)			
such as tuna, halibut, red snapper, swordfish, grouper			
mahi mahi, orange roughy, shark	varies	varies	4
Poultry (4 ounces)	196	87	4
Beef, all varieties	varies	varies	0
Pork, all varieties	varies	varies	0
Lamb, all varieties	varies	varies	0
Hot dogs (1 item)	137	504	0
Pork Sausage (4 ounces)	390	1369	0
Turkey Sausage (4 ounces)	179	1052	0
Cold cuts, all varieties	varies	varies	0
Beef jerky (2 ounces)	232	1012	0

DESSERT ITEMS

	CALORIES	SODIUM	NUT. IQ
Dark chocolate, 80-100% cocoa (1.5 ounces)	255	9	7
Cocoa Powder, unsweetened (2 tablespoons)	24	2	7
Dark chocolate, 65-79% cocoa (1.5 ounces)	246	4	6
Milk chocolate and other dark chocolate	235	35	0
Cookies made with white flour and white sugar	varies	varies	0

	CALORIES	SODIUM	NUT. IQ
Cakes and Pies made with white flour and white sugar	varies	varies	0

FAST FOODS AND SNACKS

	CALORIES	SODIUM	NUT. IQ
Potato chips (1 ounce)	154	136	0
Corn chips (1 ounce)	147	155	0
Popcorn (4 cups)	257	466	0
Pretzels (1 ounce)	108	385	0
Cheese Pizza (2 slices)	483	1354	0
Fast Food Hamburger (1 item)	265	532	0
Fast Food Cheeseburger (1 item)	313	745	0
Fast food fish sandwich (1 item)	391	689	0
Fast food chicken sandwich (1 item)	524	1178	0
Bacon, Egg and Cheese Biscuit (1 item)	432	1225	0
Chicken nuggets (4 pieces)	170	330	0
Chicken or beef tacos (2 tacos)	340	620	0
Chicken or beef burritos (1 item)	490	1250	0
French fries (1 medium serving)	370	266	0
Milk shake (12 fl oz)	419	142	0

CHAPTER SEVEN

HIGH-NUTRIENT MENUS

Earlier, we discussed my three levels of nutritional excellence. In this chapter, we will do a sample menu comparison of Nutritarian against Standard American Diet for each of the three levels.

All items with an asterisk appear in Chapter Eight, High Nutrient Recipes, beginning on page 75.

LEVEL ONE SMART

Standard American Diet	Nutritarian Diet
BREAKFAST	**BREAKFAST**
Orange juice	Fresh squeezed orange juice
Cheerios	Apple Pie Oatmeal*
Whole milk	
LUNCH	**LUNCH**
Ham and cheese sandwich with mayonnaise	Avocado Toast with Sliced Tomatoes and Toasted Pumpkin Seeds*
Apple	Baked Sweet Potato Fries*
Potato chips	Grapes
Coke	Water
DINNER	**DINNER**
Salad with bottled Italian Dressing	Salad with bottled no-oil dressing
Spaghetti and meatballs	Bean Pasta with Cashew Alfredo Sauce*
Chocolate ice cream	Steamed Asparagus *
	Chocolate Cherry Ice Cream*

NUTRITIONAL ANALYSIS

	SAD	Nutritarian
Nutrient IQ Score	**176**	**663**
Calories	2259	2050
Protein (g)	70	67
Carbohydrate (g)	327	331
Fat (g)	82	65
Cholesterol (mg)	160	0
Saturated fat (g)	30	10
Fiber (g)	24	49
Sodium (mg)	3039	1143
Vitamin C (mg)	167	198
B1, thiamine (mg)	2.4	5.0
B6, pyridoxine (mg)	2.0	2.3
Iron (mg)	28	25
Folate (mg)	1101	775
Magnesium (mg)	300	638
Calcium (mg)	1039	487
Zinc (mg)	16	12
Selenium (mcg)	137	62
Alpha tocopherol (mcg)	5.0	6.8
Beta carotene (mcg)	5427	18151
Alpha Carotene (mcg)	83	185
Lutein & Zeaxanthin (mcg)	2763	4253
Lycopene (mcg)	1582	3166

LEVEL TWO
BRILLIANT

Standard American Diet	Nutritarian Diet
BREAKFAST	BREAKFAST
Blueberry muffin	Blueberry Banana Cobbler*
Coffee with cream	
LUNCH	LUNCH
Cheeseburger on a bun	Teff Burgers* on a whole grain bun
French fries	Shredded Cabbage Slaw*
Ice tea	Watermelon
DINNER	Water
Fried chicken	DINNER
Cole slaw	Big Salad (romaine, arugula, tomato and red onion) with Almond Vinaigrette Dressing*
Corn	
Roll	Black Bean Quinoa Soup*
Cookies	Steamed broccoli
	Nutritarian Chocolate Chip Cookies*

NUTRITIONAL ANALYSIS

	SAD	Nutritarian
Nutrient IQ Score	139	878
Calories	2335	2016
Protein (g)	87	83
Carbohydrate (g)	276	332
Fat (g)	102	55
Cholesterol (mg)	257	0
Saturated fat (g)	26	10
Fiber (g)	19	66
Sodium (mg)	2627	1100
Vitamin C (mg)	31	275
B1, thiamine (mg)	1.5	4.5
B6, pyridoxine (mg)	1.5	2.6
Iron (mg)	14	25
Folate (mg)	348	897
Magnesium (mg)	186	770
Calcium (mg)	515	678
Zinc (mg)	9	13
Selenium (mcg)	117	90
Alpha tocopherol (mcg)	4.5	16.1
Beta carotene (mcg)	82	14645
Alpha Carotene (mcg)	28	1814
Lutein & Zeaxanthin (mcg)	1174	15329
Lycopene (mcg)	0	14440

LEVEL THREE GENIUS

Standard American Diet	Nutritarian Diet
BREAKFAST	**BREAKFAST**
Bagel with cream cheese	Green Apple Ginger Smoothie*
Caramel Latte	Mixed fruit cup topped with walnuts
LUNCH	**LUNCH**
Cobb Salad (with lettuce, tomato, bacon, avocado, chicken, hard-boiled egg and blue cheese	Big Salad (mixed greens, shredded cabbage, tomato and red onion) and Creamy Avocado Dressing*
Diet soda	Two Bean Chili*
DINNER	Sliced mango
Rib eye steak	**DINNER**
Baked potato with sour cream	Mushroom and White Bean Loaf*
Green beans	Cauliflower Spinach Mashed Potatoes*
Apple pie with vanilla ice cream	Kale sautéed with garlic
	Chia Pudding with fresh raspberries*

NUTRITIONAL ANALYSIS

	SAD	Nutritarian
Nutrient IQ Score	**208**	**1340**
Calories	3003	1952
Protein (g)	105	73
Carbohydrate (g)	248	303
Fat (g)	180	69
Cholesterol (mg)	680	0
Saturated fat (g)	74	15
Fiber (g)	18	83
Sodium (mg)	2327	432
Vitamin C (mg)	48	572
B1, thiamine (mg)	1.3	3.3
B6, pyridoxine (mg)	2.2	3.5
Iron (mg)	16	28
Folate (mg)	545	1162
Magnesium (mg)	226	845
Calcium (mg)	1079	1159
Zinc (mg)	13	13
Selenium (mcg)	113	46
Alpha tocopherol (mcg)	8.5	10.3
Beta carotene (mcg)	4622	27961
Alpha Carotene (mcg)	70	689
Lutein & Zeaxanthin (mcg)	3098	48088
Lycopene (mcg)	1312	7201

CHAPTER EIGHT

HIGH-NUTRIENT RECIPES

My high-nutrient recipes are among the most healthful in the world. And they taste great! The recipes that follow are just a sampling to get you started. You can find many more delicious recipes on my website, www.DrFuhrman.com. The member center on the website has over 1,700 recipes which are rated and commented on by members.

Feel free to adjust or add herbs and spices to suit your tastes – just don't add salt. Nutrient IQ Scores are given in convenient kitchen measures and are not necessarily recommended serving amounts. Adjust the scores based the size of your serving.

SMOOTHIES AND JUICES

<u>BLUEBERRY ORANGE SMOOTHIE</u> *Serves 1*

- 1 orange, peeled and seeded
- 1/2 banana (see note)
- 1/2 cup frozen blueberries
- 1 tablespoon ground flax seeds
- 2 cups chopped kale or romaine lettuce

Blend all ingredients together in a high-powered blender until smooth and creamy.

Note: Peel and freeze the other half of the banana and use for another smoothie or a Nutritarian ice cream.

NUTRIENT IQ POINTS: 137 per cup

CALORIES 265; PROTEIN 8g; CARBOHYDRATES 56g; SUGARS 26g; TOTAL FAT 4.8g; SATURATED FAT 0.5g; SODIUM 62mg; FIBER 11.3g; BETA-CAROTENE 12522ug; VITAMIN C 251mg; CALCIUM 268mg; IRON 3.2mg; FOLATE 110ug; MAGNESIUM 108mg; POTASSIUM 1141mg; ZINC 1.1mg; SELENIUM 3.7ug

CHOCOLATE PEANUT BUTTER SMOOTHIE   *Serves: 1*

2 cups chopped kale

1 tablespoon no-oil, no-salt-added peanut butter

1 tablespoon unsweetened cocoa powder

1/2 ripe frozen banana

1/2-1 cup unsweetened soy, hemp or almond milk

1/4 teaspoon pure vanilla bean powder or alcohol-free vanilla extract

Blend all ingredients in high-powered blender.

Adjust the amount of non-dairy milk to desired consistency. For added sweetness, add 1-2 pitted dates.

NUTRIENT IQ POINTS: 75 per cup

CALORIES 269; PROTEIN 14g; CARBOHYDRATES 35g; SUGARS 9g; TOTAL FAT 11.9g; SATURATED FAT 2.5g; SODIUM 107mg; FIBER 7.6g; BETA-CAROTENE 12378ug; VITAMIN C 166mg; CALCIUM 351mg; IRON 4mg; FOLATE 64ug; MAGNESIUM 133mg; POTASSIUM 1145mg; ZINC 2mg; SELENIUM 3.5ug

GREEN APPLE GINGER SMOOTHIE   *Serves: 1*

1 medium cucumber, peeled

1 ½ cups chopped kale

1 green apple, peeled and cored

1 tablespoon ground flax seeds

1 tablespoon fresh lemon juice

1 inch piece ginger, or to taste

ice

Place ingredients in a high-powered blender and blend until smooth.

NUTRIENT IQ POINTS: 203 per cup

CALORIES 197; PROTEIN 6g; CARBOHYDRATES 39g; SUGARS 20g; TOTAL FAT 4g; SATURATED FAT 0.4g; SODIUM 50mg; FIBER 7.6g; BETA-CAROTENE 9362ug; VITAMIN C 140mg; CALCIUM 192mg; IRON 2.7mg; FOLATE 67ug; MAGNESIUM 96mg; POTASSIUM 965mg; ZINC 1mg; SELENIUM 2.9ug

GO-TO GREEN JUICE   *Serves: 2*

2 cucumbers

2 large carrots

10 organic kale leaves

1 green apple, cored and cut in quarters

1 lemon, peeled

Wash all ingredients. Run all ingredients through a juicer.

NUTRIENT IQ POINTS: 116 per cup

CALORIES 152; PROTEIN 8g; CARBOHYDRATES 33g; SUGARS 16g; TOTAL FAT 1.9g; SATURATED FAT 0.2g; SODIUM 112mg; BETA-CAROTENE 19694ug; VITAMIN C 228mg; CALCIUM 283mg; IRON 3.7mg; FOLATE 100ug; MAGNESIUM 98mg; POTASSIUM 1360mg; ZINC 1.3mg; SELENIUM 1.8ug

BREAKFASTS

APPLE PIE OATMEAL   *Serves 1*

1/2 cup old fashioned or steel cut oats (see note)

1 cup water

1 apple, peeled, cored, and diced

1/4 teaspoon ground cinnamon

2 regular or 1 Medjool date, pitted, finely chopped
or 2 tablespoons raisins (optional)

2 tablespoons chopped walnuts

1/4 teaspoon pure vanilla bean powder or alcohol-free
vanilla extract

Place oats and water in small pot and bring to gentle boil.
Reduce heat to low and simmer for 5 minutes.

Stir in apples, ground cinnamon, and chopped dates
or raisins. Add additional water if needed to adjust
consistency. When oatmeal and apples are heated
through, remove from heat and stir in walnuts and
vanilla.

Note: If using steel cut oats, double the amount of water
and simmer for 20 minutes or until tender.

NUTRIENT IQ POINTS: 46 per cup

CALORIES 284; PROTEIN 7g; CARBOHYDRATES 49g; SUGARS 17g; TOTAL FAT
8.4g; SATURATED FAT 1g; SODIUM 10mg; FIBER 7g; BETA-CAROTENE 29ug;
VITAMIN C 7mg; CALCIUM 30mg; IRON 10.4mg; FOLATE 8ug; MAGNESIUM 22mg;
POTASSIUM 185mg; ZINC 0.4mg; SELENIUM 0.4ug

BERRY YOGURT   *Serves 2*

2 cups fresh or frozen blueberries, blackberries
or strawberries

3/4 cup unsweetened soy, almond or hemp milk

2 tablespoons ground flax or chia seeds

4 regular or 2 Medjool dates, pitted

Add all ingredients to high-powered blender and blend
until smooth. Chill before serving.

May be served over fresh or thawed frozen berries.

NUTRIENT IQ POINTS: 48 per cup

CALORIES 238; PROTEIN 6g; CARBOHYDRATES 47g; SUGARS 34g; TOTAL FAT
5.1g; SATURATED FAT 0.5g; SODIUM 51mg; FIBER 7.5g; BETA-CAROTENE 71ug;
VITAMIN C 14mg; CALCIUM 65mg; IRON 1.6mg; FOLATE 35ug; MAGNESIUM 72mg;
POTASSIUM 446mg; ZINC 0.8mg; SELENIUM 6.3ug

BLUEBERRY BANANA BREAKFAST COBBLER *Serves 2*

1 banana, sliced

1 cup frozen blueberries

1/4 cup old fashioned rolled oats

1 tablespoon dried currants

1/8 teaspoon pure vanilla bean powder or alcohol-free vanilla extract

2 tablespoons chopped raw almonds

2 tablespoons unsweetened, shredded coconut

1/4 teaspoon cinnamon

Combine banana, berries, oats, currants and vanilla in a microwave-safe dish. Microwave for 2 minutes. Top with almonds, coconut and cinnamon and microwave for 1 minute. Serve warm.

NUTRIENT IQ POINTS: 65 per cup

CALORIES 216; PROTEIN 4g; CARBOHYDRATES 36g; SUGARS 17g; TOTAL FAT 8.1g; SATURATED FAT 3.7g; SODIUM 4mg; FIBER 6.8g; BETA-CAROTENE 39ug; VITAMIN C 7mg; CALCIUM 34mg; IRON 3.4mg; FOLATE 21ug; MAGNESIUM 43mg; POTASSIUM 368mg; ZINC 0.5mg; SELENIUM 1.9ug

BERRY YOGURT   *Serves 2*

> 2 cups fresh or frozen blueberries, blackberries or strawberries
>
> 3/4 cup unsweetened soy, almond or hemp milk
>
> 2 tablespoons ground flax or chia seeds
>
> 4 regular or 2 Medjool dates, pitted

Add all ingredients to high-powered blender and blend until smooth. Chill before serving.

May be served over fresh or thawed frozen berries.

NUTRIENT IQ POINTS: 48 per cup

CALORIES 238; PROTEIN 6g; CARBOHYDRATES 47g; SUGARS 34g; TOTAL FAT 5.1g; SATURATED FAT 0.5g; SODIUM 51mg; FIBER 7.5g; BETA-CAROTENE 71ug; VITAMIN C 14mg; CALCIUM 65mg; IRON 1.6mg; FOLATE 35ug; MAGNESIUM 72mg; POTASSIUM 446mg; ZINC 0.8mg; SELENIUM 6.3ug

QUICK BREAKFAST QUINOA BOWL   *Serves 4*

1 cup dry quinoa

2 cups water

1 medium apple, cored and diced

1/2 cup raw almonds, chopped

1 cup fresh or thawed frozen blueberries

1/2 cup raisins or chopped, pitted dates

1 teaspoon cinnamon

1/2 cup unsweetened soy, hemp or almond milk

Place quinoa and water in a saucepan, bring to a boil, cover, reduce heat, and simmer for 15 minutes or until quinoa is tender and all the water is absorbed. Fluff with a fork.

Add remaining ingredients and cook for another 2-3 minutes, stirring frequently. Divide among four bowls

NUTRIENT IQ POINTS: 46 per cup

CALORIES 332; PROTEIN 10g; CARBOHYDRATES 57g; SUGARS 20g; TOTAL FAT 9.1g; SATURATED FAT 0.8g; SODIUM 33mg; FIBER 7.8g; BETA-CAROTENE 30ug; VITAMIN C 4mg; CALCIUM 140mg; IRON 3mg; FOLATE 90ug; MAGNESIUM 129mg; POTASSIUM 539mg; ZINC 1.8mg; SELENIUM 4.1ug

SCRAMBLED TOFU WITH RED PEPPER, TOMATO AND SPINACH *Serves 2*

3 scallions, diced

1/2 cup finely chopped red bell pepper

1 medium tomato, chopped

2 cloves garlic, minced or pressed

14 ounces firm tofu, drained and crumbled

1 tablespoon Dr. Fuhrman's MatoZest or other no-salt seasoning blend, adjusted to taste

1 tablespoon nutritional yeast

5 ounces baby spinach, coarsely chopped

1 teaspoon coconut aminos

In a large skillet, over medium/high heat, sauté scallions, red pepper, tomato, and garlic in 1/4 cup water for 5 minutes. Add remaining ingredients and cook for another 5 minutes.

If desired, serve with Dr. Fuhrman's no-salt, no-sugar Ketchup.

NUTRIENT IQ POINTS: 102 per cup

CALORIES 249; PROTEIN 24g; CARBOHYDRATES 19g; SUGARS 6g; TOTAL FAT 9.7g; SATURATED FAT 1.1g; SODIUM 148mg; FIBER 6.7g; BETA-CAROTENE 5003ug; VITAMIN C 84mg; CALCIUM 367mg; IRON 5.7mg; FOLATE 194ug; MAGNESIUM 86mg; POTASSIUM 694mg; ZINC 1.6mg; SELENIUM 1.6ug

SOUPS AND STEWS

Serves 4

1 medium onion, chopped

1 green bell pepper, chopped

1 large carrot, chopped

4 cloves garlic, minced

1 cup chopped fresh tomato

1 teaspoon ground cumin

2 teaspoons chili powder

1/4 teaspoon crushed red pepper flakes

5 cups low-sodium or no-salt-added vegetable broth

1/2 cup quinoa, rinsed

3 cups cooked black beans or 2 (15 ounce) cans low-sodium or no-salt-added black beans, drained

4 cups spinach or thinly sliced kale

1/4 cup chopped cilantro

1 tablespoon fresh lime juice

1 avocado, chopped

In a soup pot, combine onion, green pepper, carrots, garlic, tomatoes, cumin, chili powder, red pepper flakes and vegetable broth. Bring to a boil, reduce heat and cook for 5 minutes. Stir in quinoa, cover and cook for 10 minutes. Add black beans and continue cooking until heated through and quinoa is tender, about 10 minutes. Add spinach or kale and stir until wilted.

Remove from heat and stir in cilantro and lime juice. Serve garnished with chopped avocado.

NUTRIENT IQ POINTS: 79 per cup

CALORIES 372; PROTEIN 19g; CARBOHYDRATES 65g; SUGARS 4g; TOTAL FAT 5.6g; SATURATED FAT 0.8g; SODIUM 244mg; FIBER 17.9g; BETA-CAROTENE 8221ug; VITAMIN C 118mg; CALCIUM 203mg; IRON 6.4mg; FOLATE 286ug; MAGNESIUM 178mg; POTASSIUM 1279mg; ZINC 2.8mg; SELENIUM 4.9ug

CREAMY MUSHROOM SOUP   *Serves 4*

20 ounces white or brown mushrooms, sliced

1 cup carrot juice

2 cups no-salt-added or low-sodium vegetable broth

1 large sweet onion

2 small carrots, sliced

2 tablespoons Dr.Fuhrman's Vegizest or other no-salt seasoning blend, adjusted to taste

1 1/2 teaspoons coconut aminos

4 cloves garlic, pressed

2 tablespoons fresh cilantro

1 cup walnuts

2 cups unsweetened soy, hemp or almond milk

1/4 teaspoon black pepper, or to taste

Combine all ingredients except cilantro, walnuts, non-dairy milk and black pepper in a large pot. Cook about 25 minutes or until carrots and mushrooms are tender. Remove from heat and stir in fresh cilantro.

Pour 3/4 of the soup in a high-powered blender with the walnuts and non-dairy milk. Blend until smooth. Pour mixture back into pan, stir and heat through. Season with black pepper.

NUTRIENT IQ POINTS: 79 per cup

CALORIES 331; PROTEIN 12g; CARBOHYDRATES 30g; SUGARS 12g; TOTAL FAT 21.2g; SATURATED FAT 1.9g; SODIUM 291mg; FIBER 6g; BETA-CAROTENE 7585ug; VITAMIN C 18mg; CALCIUM 347mg; IRON 3.3mg; FOLATE 77ug; MAGNESIUM 97mg; POTASSIUM 1035mg; ZINC 2.1mg; SELENIUM 16.1ug

LEMON LENTIL SOUP   *Serves 4*

1 1/2 cups carrots, peeled and chopped

1 cup celery, chopped

4 cups no-salt-added or low-sodium vegetable broth

1 cup red lentils, rinsed and drained

3/4 teaspoon ground coriander

1 teaspoon ground cumin

3 tablespoons raw cashews

1/4 cup fresh lemon juice (about 2 small lemons)

1 head baby bok choy, chopped (could substitute 2 cups chopped greens, such as kale or spinach)

2 tablespoons chopped parsley

black pepper, to taste

Place carrots, celery, vegetable broth, lentils, coriander and cumin in a pot and bring to a boil. Reduce heat, cover and simmer for 40 minutes or until lentils and vegetables are tender.

In a blender or food processor, blend 1 cup of the soup with cashews and lemon juice. Return to pot along with bok choy or greens and heat until greens are wilted. Stir in parsley and season with pepper.

NUTRIENT IQ POINTS: 58 per cup

CALORIES 301; PROTEIN 22g; CARBOHYDRATES 45g; SUGARS 7g; TOTAL FAT 5.5g; SATURATED FAT 1.1g; SODIUM 268mg; FIBER 19g; BETA-CAROTENE 9787ug; VITAMIN C 109mg; CALCIUM 296mg; IRON 7mg; FOLATE 394ug; MAGNESIUM 133mg; POTASSIUM 1495mg; ZINC 3.5mg; SELENIUM 6.6ug

TOMATO FLORENTINE SOUP   *Serves 4*

1 large onion, chopped

1 celery stalk, chopped

3 garlic cloves, minced

5 cups low-sodium or no-salt-added vegetable broth

3 cups diced fresh tomatoes, undrained or 1 (26 ounce) carton diced tomatoes (see note)

6 ounces (3/4 cup) tomato paste (see note)

3 tablespoons raisins, minced

1 1/2 cups cooked great northern beans or 1 (15 ounce) can low-sodium or no-salt-added great northern beans, drained

5 ounces spinach

5 ounces baby kale

1/4 teaspoon ground black pepper, or to taste

1/4 cup nutritional yeast

6 medium fresh basil leaves, finely chopped

In a soup pot, combine onion, celery, garlic, broth, tomatoes, tomato paste, and raisins. Bring to a boil, reduce heat and simmer for about 20 minutes, stirring occasionally.

Add beans, spinach, kale, pepper, nutritional yeast, and basil. Stir to combine. Simmer until greens are wilted and soup is heated through. Additional vegetable broth can be added to adjust consistency.

Note: Select tomatoes packed in glass or cartons. These materials do not contain BPA.

NUTRIENT IQ POINTS: 88 per cup

CALORIES 248; PROTEIN 15g; CARBOHYDRATES 46g; SUGARS 15g; TOTAL FAT 1.6g; SATURATED FAT 0.3g; SODIUM 227mg; FIBER 12.2g; BETA-CAROTENE 6304ug; VITAMIN C 85mg; CALCIUM 208mg; IRON 5.7mg; FOLATE 184ug; MAGNESIUM 125mg; POTASSIUM 1511mg; ZINC 3.1mg; SELENIUM 6.3ug

TWO BEAN CHILI   *Serves 4*

1 cup chopped onion

1/2 cup chopped green bell pepper, fresh or frozen

1 clove garlic, chopped

3/4 cup water

2 tablespoons tomato paste

1 tablespoon chili powder

2 teaspoons ground cumin

1/4 teaspoon black pepper

1 1/2 cups cooked or 1 (15 ounce) can low-sodium or no-salt-added black beans, drained

3 cups cooked or 2 (15 ounce) cans low-sodium or no-salt-added red pinto or kidney beans, drained

2 cups low-sodium or no-salt-added vegetable broth

1 1/2 cups diced tomatoes

1 tablespoon yellow cornmeal

Water sauté onion and bell pepper in a soup pot until almost tender. Add garlic and cook for another minute. Stir in water, tomato paste, chili powder, cumin, black pepper, beans, vegetable broth and diced tomatoes and bring to a boil. Reduce heat, cover and simmer for 10 minutes. Stir in cornmeal and cook for an additional two minutes.

Note: If desired, 1 cup of frozen corn and/or frozen chopped broccoli may be added before soup is simmered.

NUTRIENT IQ POINTS: 88 per cup

CALORIES 317; PROTEIN 19g; CARBOHYDRATES 59g; SUGARS 6g; TOTAL FAT 1.9g; SATURATED FAT 0.3g; SODIUM 119mg; FIBER 18.6g; BETA-CAROTENE 725ug; VITAMIN C 31mg; CALCIUM 107mg; IRON 7.2mg; FOLATE 290ug; MAGNESIUM 132mg; POTASSIUM 1164mg; ZINC 2.6mg; SELENIUM 3.9ug

SALAD DRESSINGS AND SAUCES

CREAMY AVOCADO DRESSING   *Serves 4*

2 ripe avocados, peeled, pitted and chopped

2 tablespoons nutritional yeast

1/4 cup unsweetened soy, hemp or almond milk

2-3 small shallots, according to taste

1/4 cup white wine vinegar

Blend all ingredients in a high-powered blender until smooth and creamy.

You can modify amounts of shallot and non-dairy milk to adjust taste and consistency.

NUTRIENT IQ POINTS: 9 per tablespoon

CALORIES 143; PROTEIN 4g; CARBOHYDRATES 9g; SUGARS 1g; TOTAL FAT 10.9g; SATURATED FAT 1.5g; SODIUM 14mg; FIBER 5.8g; BETA-CAROTENE 43ug; VITAMIN C 7mg; CALCIUM 35mg; IRON 0.8mg; FOLATE 64ug; MAGNESIUM 30mg; POTASSIUM 397mg; ZINC 1.4mg; SELENIUM 0.5ug

ALMOND VINAIGRETTE DRESSING   *Serves 6*

1 cup unsweetened soy, hemp or almond milk

3/4 cup raw almonds

2 tablespoons hemp seeds

1/4 cup balsamic vinegar

2 tablespoons fresh lemon juice

1/4 cup raisins

2 teaspoons Dijon mustard

1 clove garlic

Blend ingredients in a high-powered blender until creamy and smooth.

NUTRIENT IQ POINTS: 4 per tablespoon

CALORIES 181; PROTEIN 7g; CARBOHYDRATES 13g; SUGARS 6g; TOTAL FAT 12.5g; SATURATED FAT 1g; SODIUM 38mg; FIBER 3.4g; BETA-CAROTENE 1ug; VITAMIN C 2mg; CALCIUM 122mg; IRON 1.3mg; FOLATE 13ug; MAGNESIUM 75mg; POTASSIUM 284mg; ZINC 0.9mg; SELENIUM 1.3ug

ORANGE SESAME DRESSING   *Serves 4*

4 tablespoons unhulled sesame seeds, divided

2 navel oranges, peeled

1/4 cup Dr. Fuhrman's Blood Orange Vinegar or white wine vinegar

1/4 cup raw cashews

1 tablespoon lemon juice, optional

Lightly toast the sesame seeds in a dry skillet over medium high heat for about 3 minutes, shaking the pan frequently.

In a high-powered blender, combine oranges, vinegar, cashews, lemon juice, if desired and 2 tablespoons of the sesame seeds.

Toss with the salad, sprinkling remaining sesame seeds on top.

Serving Suggestion: Toss with mixed greens, shredded cabbage, tomatoes, red onions and additional diced oranges or kiwi.

NUTRIENT IQ POINTS: 4 per tablespoon

CALORIES 137; PROTEIN 4g; CARBOHYDRATES 14g; SUGARS 7g; TOTAL FAT 8.3g; SATURATED FAT 1.3g; SODIUM 3mg; FIBER 2.9g; BETA-CAROTENE 61ug; VITAMIN C 43mg; CALCIUM 122mg; IRON 2mg; FOLATE 35ug; MAGNESIUM 65mg; POTASSIUM 229mg; ZINC 1.3mg; SELENIUM 4.8ug

CASHEW ALFREDO SAUCE   *Serves 4*

1 cup raw cashews

2 tablespoons unhulled sesame seeds

1 1/2 cups unsweetened soy, hemp or almond milk

3 tablespoons nutritional yeast

2 tablespoons lemon juice or more to taste

1 teaspoon Dr. Fuhrman's VegiZest or other no-salt seasoning blend, adjusted to taste

1 tablespoon chopped garlic or to taste

Blend all ingredients in a high-powered blender. Add more non-dairy milk if needed to adjust consistency. It should be fairly thick but still pour out of the blender.

Serve over steamed vegetables, bean pasta or salads.

NUTRIENT IQ POINTS: 4 per tablespoon

CALORIES 258; PROTEIN 11g; CARBOHYDRATES 15g; SUGARS 2g; TOTAL FAT 18.5g; SATURATED FAT 3g; SODIUM 78mg; FIBER 3g; VITAMIN C 4mg; CALCIUM 261mg; IRON 3.6mg; FOLATE 18ug; MAGNESIUM 132mg; POTASSIUM 262mg; ZINC 3.6mg; SELENIUM 8.7ug

SALADS

1 cup uncooked farro
10 ounces mushrooms, sliced
1/4 cup chopped red onion
3 cups baby arugula
For the Dressing:
1 medium tomato
1/3 cup raw cashews
1 tablespoon hemp seeds
1/4 cup water
1/2 lime, juiced
1 tablespoon balsamic vinegar

In a saucepan, heat 2 cups of water to boiling. Stir in farro; return to a boil. Reduce heat to low, cover and cook for 20 to 25 minutes or until farro is tender. Drain.

Meanwhile, water sauté the mushrooms until they are soft and lightly browned. Combine cooked farro, mushrooms, chopped onion and arugula.

Blend dressing ingredients together in a high-powered blender. Add desired amount of dressing to salad and toss.

Serve warm or at room temperature.

NUTRIENT IQ POINTS: 118 per cup

CALORIES 311; PROTEIN 13g; CARBOHYDRATES 47g; SUGARS 4g; TOTAL FAT 8.1g; SATURATED FAT 1.1g; SODIUM 13mg; FIBER 9.2g; BETA-CAROTENE 354ug; VITAMIN C 11mg; CALCIUM 61mg; IRON 3.5mg; FOLATE 39ug; MAGNESIUM 69mg; POTASSIUM 485mg; ZINC 1.4mg; SELENIUM 9ug

Kale and Red Cabbage Salad with Apples and Dried Cherries

Serves 2

1 bunch kale, tough stems and center ribs removed

1 avocado, peeled and chopped

2 tablespoons lemon juice

1 tablespoon white balsamic vinegar

1 cup thinly sliced red cabbage

1 large apple, cored and chopped

2 tablespoons chopped unsweetened dried cherries or raisins

1/2 medium red onion, minced

2 tablespoons chives, chopped

Roll up each kale leaf and slice thinly. Add to bowl along with avocado, lemon juice and vinegar. Using your hands, massage the avocado, lemon juice and vinegar into the kale leaves until the kale starts to soften and wilt and each leaf is coated, about 2 to 3 minutes.

Mix in red cabbage, apple, dried cherries, onion and chives.

NUTRIENT IQ POINTS: 156 per cup

CALORIES 317; PROTEIN 8g; CARBOHYDRATES 53g; SUGARS 16g; TOTAL FAT 12g; SATURATED FAT 1.7g; SODIUM 92mg; FIBER 12.4g; BETA-CAROTENE 15840ug; VITAMIN C 244mg; CALCIUM 270mg; IRON 3.9mg; FOLATE 130ug; MAGNESIUM 94mg; POTASSIUM 1372mg; ZINC 1.4mg; SELENIUM 2.2ug

Shredded Cabbage Slaw   *Serves 4*

- 1/4 small red cabbage, thinly shredded
- 1/2 small green cabbage, thinly shredded
- 1 carrot, shredded
- 1/4 cup finely chopped onion
- 1 teaspoon celery seed
- 1/2 cup raw cashews
- 2 tablespoons hemp seeds
- 1/4 cup raisins or currants
- 1/2 cup unsweetened soy, hemp or almond milk
- 2 cloves garlic
- 2 tablespoons apple cider vinegar
- 2 tablespoons lemon juice
- 1 teaspoon Dijon mustard

In a large bowl, mix together red and green cabbage, carrot, onion and celery seed.

Blend remaining ingredients in a high-powered blender.

Toss cabbage mixture with desired amount of dressing.

NUTRIENT IQ POINTS: 110 per cup

CALORIES 151; PROTEIN 5g; CARBOHYDRATES 20g; SUGARS 10g; TOTAL FAT 6.7g; SATURATED FAT 1.2g; SODIUM 57mg; FIBER 3.8g; BETA-CAROTENE 1232ug; VITAMIN C 46mg; CALCIUM 72mg; IRON 2mg; FOLATE 49ug; MAGNESIUM 67mg; POTASSIUM 433mg; ZINC 1.1mg; SELENIUM 4.9ug

THREE BEAN MANGO SALAD   *Serves 6*

1 1/2 cups cooked or 1 (15 ounce) can no-salt-added or low-sodium cannellini beans, drained

1 1/2 cups cooked or 1 (15 ounce) can no-salt-added or low-sodium kidney beans, drained

1 1/2 cups cooked or 1 (15 ounce) can no-salt-added or low-sodium chickpeas, drained

2 mangoes, peeled, pitted and cubed

1/2 red onion, finely chopped

1/2 red bell pepper, chopped

1/2 cup finely chopped flat leaf parsley

10 ounces mixed baby greens

For the Dressing

1/2 cup water

1/3 cup cider vinegar

1/4 cup raw almonds

1/4 cup raisins

2 teaspoons whole grain mustard

1/2 teaspoon dried oregano

In a large bowl, mix the beans, mangoes, onion, bell pepper and parsley.

Blend water, vinegar, almonds, raisins, mustard and oregano in a high-powered blender until smooth. Add dressing to bean mixture and toss to coat.

Chill in the refrigerator for several hours, to allow beans to soak up the flavor of the dressing.

Serve on top of the mixed greens.

NUTRIENT IQ POINTS: 86 per cup

CALORIES 328; PROTEIN 16g; CARBOHYDRATES 59g; SUGARS 23g; TOTAL FAT 5.1g; SATURATED FAT 0.6g; SODIUM 50mg; FIBER 12.5g; BETA-CAROTENE 3912ug; VITAMIN C 69mg; CALCIUM 153mg; IRON 5.7mg; FOLATE 280ug; MAGNESIUM 119mg; POTASSIUM 1065mg; ZINC 2.4mg; SELENIUM 4.4ug

MAIN DISHES

Avocado Toast with Sliced Tomatoes
and Toasted Pumpkin Seeds   *Serves 2*

  2 (100% whole grain) pitas, lightly toasted
  1 ripe avocado, mashed
  1 medium tomato, sliced
  1/2 red onion, sliced thinly
  2 tablespoons raw pumpkin seeds, toasted (see note)
  black pepper or crushed red pepper flakes, to taste

Spread the mashed avocado on top of the toasted pitas. Add tomato slices and sliced onion and sprinkle with pumpkin seeds. Season with your choice of ground black pepper or red pepper flakes.

Note: Other seeds or chopped nuts may be substituted.

NUTRIENT IQ POINTS: 132 per one pita

CALORIES 267; PROTEIN 8g; CARBOHYDRATES 30g; SUGARS 3g; TOTAL FAT 15g; SATURATED FAT 2.2g; SODIUM 120mg; FIBER 9.2g; BETA-CAROTENE 1571ug; VITAMIN C 16mg; CALCIUM 23mg; IRON 2.4mg; FOLATE 78ug; MAGNESIUM 76mg; POTASSIUM 583mg; ZINC 1.2mg; SELENIUM 1.1ug

Broccoli and Shiitake Mushrooms with
Thai Peanut Sauce   *Serves 4*

For the Thai Peanut Sauce (see note):

1 1/2 cups water

7 regular or 3 1/2 Medjool dates, pitted

1/3 cup no-oil, no-salt peanut butter

2 tablespoons unsweetened shredded coconut

1 teaspoon minced ginger

1 tablespoon lime juice

1 teaspoon red curry powder

1/2 teaspoon chili powder

1/2 teaspoon ground cumin

1/4 teaspoon ground turmeric

For the Vegetables:

1 cup chopped onions

6 cups broccoli florets

1 cup thinly sliced red bell pepper strips

2 cups trimmed snow peas

2 cups sliced shiitake mushrooms

To make the sauce:

Blend water and dates in a high-powered blender, then add peanut butter, coconut, ginger, lime juice and spices and blend again until smooth and well-combined.

To cook the vegetables:

Heat 1/4 cup water in a large non-stick wok or skillet, then add chopped onions and broccoli, cover and cook for 4 minutes stirring occasionally and adding additional water as needed to prevent sticking. Remove cover and add red bell pepper strips, shiitake mushrooms and snow peas and cook for an additional 4 minutes or until vegetables are crisp-tender. Add desired amount of sauce and continue to stir fry for 1-2 minutes to heat through.

Note: In a rush? Dr. Fuhrman's time-saving bottled sauces are available at www.drfuhrman.com. Thai Curry Sauce would work well in this recipe.

NUTRIENT IQ POINTS: 78 per cup

CALORIES 295; PROTEIN 13g; CARBOHYDRATES 39g; SUGARS 18g; TOTAL FAT 13.5g; SATURATED FAT 3.2g; SODIUM 70mg; FIBER 11.4g; BETA-CAROTENE 1123ug; VITAMIN C 174mg; CALCIUM 117mg; IRON 3.4mg; FOLATE 151ug; MAGNESIUM 111mg; POTASSIUM 1152mg; ZINC 2.6mg; SELENIUM 11.9ug

Cauliflower, Spinach Mashed "Potatoes" *Serves 4*

6 cups fresh or frozen cauliflower florets
2-4 cloves garlic, sliced
10 ounces fresh spinach
1/2 cup raw cashew butter
2 tablespoons hemp seeds
1 teaspoon Dr. Fuhrman's VegiZest or other no-salt
seasoning blend, adjusted to taste
1/4 teaspoon nutmeg
unsweetened soy, almond or hemp milk, as needed

Steam cauliflower and garlic about 8 to 10 minutes or until tender. Drain and press out as much water as possible in strainer. Place in a high-powered blender or food processor.

Steam spinach until just wilted and set aside.

Blend cauliflower, garlic, cashew butter, hemp seeds, VegiZest and nutmeg until smooth and creamy. Add non-dairy milk if needed to adjust consistency. Stir in wilted spinach.

NUTRIENT IQ POINTS: 181 per cup

CALORIES 250; PROTEIN 11g; CARBOHYDRATES 20g; SUGARS 3g; TOTAL FAT 16.6g; SATURATED FAT 3.3g; SODIUM 110mg; FIBER 5.6g; BETA-CAROTENE 3987ug; VITAMIN C 98mg; CALCIUM 125mg; IRON 4.3mg; FOLATE 253ug; MAGNESIUM 165mg; POTASSIUM 1057mg; ZINC 2.5mg; SELENIUM 5.6ug

Collard Greens and Beans   *Serves 2*

1 large onion, sliced

3 cloves garlic, thinly sliced

1 bunch collard greens, stems removed and cut into
1/2 inch strips

1/4 teaspoon red pepper flakes or more to taste

1/2 cup low-sodium or no-salt-added vegetable broth

1 1/2 cups cooked or 1 (15 ounce) can low-sodium or
no-salt-added cannellini beans

1 1/2 cups chopped tomato

2 tablespoons lemon juice

Heat 2-3 tablespoons water in a large sauté pan or wok and
water sauté onion and garlic until tender. Add collards,
red pepper flakes and vegetable broth, cover, and cook for
5 minutes. Add beans, tomatoes and lemon juice, cover
and continue cooking for an additional 5 minutes or until
collards are wilted and tender. Add additional vegetable
broth if needed to prevent sticking.

NUTRIENT IQ POINTS: 166 per cup

CALORIES 276; PROTEIN 17g; CARBOHYDRATES 53g; SUGARS 8g; TOTAL FAT
1.2g; SATURATED FAT 0.2g; SODIUM 67mg; FIBER 14.9g; BETA-CAROTENE
3379ug; VITAMIN C 57mg; CALCIUM 270mg; IRON 5.8mg; FOLATE 264ug;
MAGNESIUM 116mg; POTASSIUM 1341mg; ZINC 2.4mg; SELENIUM 3.7ug

Mushroom and White Bean Loaf *Serves 8*

1 large sweet potato

1 medium onion, finely chopped

2 stalks celery, finely chopped

1 medium carrot, finely chopped

2 cloves garlic, finely chopped

2 cups finely chopped mushrooms

1 1/2 cups cooked or 1 (15 ounce) can no-salt-added or low-sodium cannellini beans, drained

8 ounces extra firm tofu, excess water squeezed out

1/4 cup low-sodium ketchup plus additional for top of loaf

1 tablespoon Dr. Fuhrman's MatoZest or other no-salt seasoning blend, adjusted to taste

1 tablespoon mustard

1/2 teaspoon poultry seasoning (a blend of sage, thyme, marjoram, rosemary, black pepper and nutmeg)

1/2 teaspoon oregano

1/4 teaspoon black pepper

1 cup old fashioned oats, pulsed in food processor to a coarse powder

1/2 cup chopped pecans

1/4 cup chopped parsley

Pierce sweet potato in several places with a fork and microwave until soft, about 5-6 minutes. When cool enough to handle, peel and set aside.

Heat a large skillet. Add the onion, celery, carrot, garlic and mushrooms and cook, stirring regularly until tender and all the water from the mushrooms has evaporated. Mash beans with a fork and add to the mushroom mixture.

Place the peeled sweet potato into a food processor along with the tofu, ketchup, MatoZest, mustard, poultry seasoning, oregano and black pepper. Process until smooth and well combined.

Add tofu mixture to mushrooms and beans along with oats, pecans and parsley and mix well.

Spoon into a loaf pan that has been lightly rubbed with a minimal amount of oil. Spread ketchup on top. Bake at 350 degrees for 1 hour and 10 minutes. Allow to sit for 30 minutes before slicing.

NUTRIENT IQ POINTS: 69 per slice (8 slices/loaf)

CALORIES 217; PROTEIN 11g; CARBOHYDRATES 27g; SUGARS 4g; TOTAL FAT 8.6g; SATURATED FAT 1g; SODIUM 60mg; FIBER 7.6g; BETA-CAROTENE 2201ug; VITAMIN C 7mg; CALCIUM 256mg; IRON 5mg; FOLATE 80ug; MAGNESIUM 63mg; POTASSIUM 519mg; ZINC 1.5mg; SELENIUM 11.4ug

Portobello Pizza   *Serves 1*

2 large Portobello mushrooms, stems removed
1/4 teaspoon garlic powder
1/4 teaspoon dried basil
1/4 teaspoon dried oregano
1/2 cup low-sodium pasta sauce
1/3 cup thinly sliced onion
1/3 cup thinly sliced green or red bell pepper
2-3 tablespoons Nutritarian Parmesan **(see note)**

Preheat oven to 350 degrees F.

Place mushrooms on a parchment-lined baking sheet, gill side up and sprinkle with garlic powder, basil and oregano. Bake for 6 minutes.

Top with tomato sauce, onions and peppers and a sprinkle of Nutritarian Parmesan. Bake for an additional 20 minutes or until vegetables are tender.

Note: To make Nutritarian Parmesan, place 1/4 cup walnuts or almonds and 1/4 cup nutritional yeast in a food processor and pulse until the texture of grated Parmesan is achieved. Store in an airtight container and refrigerate.

NUTRIENT IQ POINTS: 106 per mushroom

CALORIES 179; PROTEIN 11g; CARBOHYDRATES 26g; SUGARS 14g; TOTAL FAT 4.7g; SATURATED FAT 0.6g; CHOLESTEROL 2.6mg; SODIUM 59mg; FIBER 8g; BETA-CAROTENE 569ug; VITAMIN C 30mg; CALCIUM 79mg; IRON 2.6mg; FOLATE 78ug; MAGNESIUM 54mg; POTASSIUM 1178mg; ZINC 3mg; SELENIUM 33.2ug

Seasoned Sweet Potato Fries   *Serves 4*

2 tablespoons water
1/2 teaspoon coconut aminos
1/2 teaspoon dried thyme
1/2 teaspoon dried oregano
1/2 teaspoon dried basil
1/2 teaspoon paprika
2 tablespoons nutritional yeast
freshly ground black pepper, to taste
2 large sweet potatoes, peeled and cut into fry shapes
or long wedges

Preheat oven to 375 degrees F.

In a large mixing bowl, whisk together the water, coconut aminos, dried herbs, paprika, nutritional yeast and pepper. Add the sweet potatoes and toss until thoroughly coated.

Place the sweet potatoes in a single layer on a Silpat-lined or non-stick baking sheet and bake for 45 minutes or until baked through and lightly browned, giving them a stir every 15 minutes.

NUTRIENT IQ POINTS: 45 per potato

CALORIES 74; PROTEIN 3g; CARBOHYDRATES 15g; SUGARS 3g; TOTAL FAT 0.3g; SATURATED FAT 0.1g; SODIUM 54mg; FIBER 3.1g; BETA-CAROTENE 5613ug; VITAMIN C 2mg; CALCIUM 34mg; IRON 1.1mg; FOLATE 9ug; MAGNESIUM 24mg; POTASSIUM 235mg; ZINC 1mg; SELENIUM 0.4ug

Spiced Butternut and Brussels Bowl   *Serves 4*

12 ounces butternut squash, cut into 1/2 inch cubes
1 orange, juiced
pinch ground cinnamon
pinch ground cloves
pinch ground allspice
pinch cayenne pepper
1 large shallot, chopped
3/4 pound Brussel sprouts, shredded or very thinly sliced
1/4 cup toasted pecans, chopped
2 tablespoons currants or raisins
2 tablespoons balsamic vinegar
1/2 teaspoon fresh thyme, chopped
ground black pepper, to taste

Preheat oven to 350 degrees.

Mix the squash with the orange juice, cinnamon, cloves, allspice and cayenne. Place the mixture in a baking pan, cover with foil and roast until tender and caramelized but still firm when a fork is inserted, about 20 minutes.

Meanwhile, heat 2 tablespoons water in a large skillet and sauté shallot for 1 minute, add shredded Brussels sprouts and cook for 2-3 minutes, until warm and slightly wilted.

Add a small amount of additional water if needed to prevent from sticking.

Place roasted butternut squash and sautéed Brussels sprouts in a bowl and toss with pecans, currants, vinegar and thyme. Season with black pepper.

NUTRIENT IQ POINTS: 105 per cup

CALORIES 158; PROTEIN 5g; CARBOHYDRATES 28g; SUGARS 11g; TOTAL FAT 4.9g; SATURATED FAT 0.5g; SODIUM 28mg; FIBER 6.2g; BETA-CAROTENE 4006ug; VITAMIN C 106mg; CALCIUM 95mg; IRON 2.3mg; FOLATE 88ug; MAGNESIUM 64mg; POTASSIUM 788mg; ZINC 0.8mg; SELENIUM 2.2ug

Teff Burgers *Serves 8*

2 cups water
2/3 cup teff (see note)
1 cup minced onion
1 cup minced mushrooms
1 medium carrot, grated
1 cup finely chopped kale
1 teaspoon cumin
1 teaspoon chili powder
1/2 teaspoon garlic powder
1/4 teaspoon black pepper
1 1/2 cups cooked or 1 (15 ounce) can no-salt-added or low-sodium red kidney beans, drained
1/4 cup unfortified nutritional yeast

Preheat oven to 350 degrees F.

In a saucepan with a cover, bring water to a boil, stir in teff, reduce to a simmer, cover and cook for 15 minutes or until water is absorbed and teff is tender, stirring occasionally.

In a sauté pan, heat 2 tablespoons of water, add onion and sauté until starting to become translucent, adding more water if needed. Add mushrooms, carrot and kale and cook until mushrooms have released their liquid and the carrots and kale are soft. Stir in cumin, chili powder, garlic powder and black pepper and cook for an additional minute.

Place the beans in a mixing bowl and mash with a fork. Stir in the cooked teff, sautéed vegetables and the nutritional yeast.

Divide the mixture into 8 burgers and place on a parchment or silpat-lined baking pan. Bake for 20 minutes, then turn and bake for an additional 15 minutes.

If desired, serve on a 100% whole grain pita with sliced onion, tomato and lettuce.

Note: Teff is a tiny whole grain with a mild, nutty flavor.

NUTRIENT IQ POINTS: 54 per burger

CALORIES 77; PROTEIN 6g; CARBOHYDRATES 13g; SUGARS 2g; TOTAL FAT 0.6g; SATURATED FAT 0.1g; SODIUM 20mg; FIBER 4.2g; BETA-CAROTENE 1457ug; VITAMIN C 13mg; CALCIUM 36mg; IRON 1.6mg; FOLATE 53ug; MAGNESIUM 29mg; POTASSIUM 267mg; ZINC 1.3mg; SELENIUM 1.5ug

DESSERTS

BANANA MANGO SORBET *Serves 2*

4 slices unsweetened, unsulfured dried mango **(see note)**
1/4 cup unsweetened soy, hemp or almond milk
1 ripe banana, frozen
2 cups frozen mango
6 ice cubes

Soak dried mango in non-dairy milk until softened, at least one hour.

Add dried mango and soaking liquid to a high-powered blender along with remaining ingredients and blend until creamy but still firm.

If desired, serve topped with walnuts or pecans.

Note: 2 medjool dates or 4 regular dates may be substituted for the dried mango.

NUTRIENT IQ POINTS: 10 per ½ cup

CALORIES 173; PROTEIN 2g; CARBOHYDRATES 43g; SUGARS 33g; TOTAL FAT 1.2g; SATURATED FAT 0.2g; SODIUM 26mg; FIBER 4.2g; BETA-CAROTENE 1223ug; VITAMIN C 65mg; CALCIUM 89mg; IRON 0.7mg; FOLATE 84ug; MAGNESIUM 37mg; POTASSIUM 570mg; ZINC 0.3mg; SELENIUM 1.7ug

CHIA PUDDING   *Serves 4*

1 cup unsweetened soy, hemp or almond milk
1/2 cup unsweetened, shredded coconut
1 cup water
2-4 medjool or 4-8 regular dates, pitted (see note)
1/2 teaspoon pure vanilla bean powder or alcohol-free vanilla extract
1/2 - 3/4 teaspoon ground cardamom
1/2 cup chia seeds, divided

Blend milk, coconut, water, dates, vanilla, cardamom and 1/4 cup of the chia seeds in a high-powered blender. Add additional milk if needed to adjust consistency. Stir in remaining 1/4 cup chia seeds. Refrigerate for 15 minutes and stir again to distribute seeds evenly.

If desired, top with fresh berries and/or toasted unsweetened coconut.

For a parfait, alternate layers of berries with pudding in a wine glass.

For a chocolate chia pudding, blend in 2 tablespoons natural cocoa powder.

Note: Adjust dates to desired sweetness.

NUTRIENT IQ POINTS: 22 per ½ cup

CALORIES 280; PROTEIN 7g; CARBOHYDRATES 34g; SUGARS 19g; TOTAL FAT 15g; SATURATED FAT 7.3g; SODIUM 42mg; FIBER 11.1g; BETA-CAROTENE 23ug; VITAMIN C 1mg; CALCIUM 171mg; IRON 2.7mg; FOLATE 16ug; MAGNESIUM 111mg; POTASSIUM 391mg; ZINC 1.4mg; SELENIUM 16.8ug

CHOCOLATE CHERRY ICE CREAM   *Serves 2*

1/2 cup unsweetened vanilla soy, hemp or almond milk
1 tablespoon natural, non-alkalized cocoa powder
4 regular dates or 2 Medjool dates, pitted
1 1/2 cups frozen dark sweet cherries
1/2 tablespoon pure vanilla bean powder or alcohol-free
vanilla extract, optional

Blend all ingredients together in a high-powered blender
or food processor until smooth and creamy.

NUTRIENT IQ POINTS: 26 per ½ cup

CALORIES 120; PROTEIN 4g; CARBOHYDRATES 26g; SUGARS 20g; TOTAL FAT
1.9g; SATURATED FAT 0.5g; SODIUM 25mg; FIBER 4.2g; BETA-CAROTENE 608ug;
VITAMIN C 2mg; CALCIUM 101mg; IRON 1.4mg; FOLATE 9ug; MAGNESIUM 40mg;
POTASSIUM 352mg; ZINC 0.6mg; SELENIUM 0.8ug

NUTRITARIAN CHOCOLATE CHIP COOKIES *Serves 10*

1 1/2 cups cooked or 1 (15 ounce) can low-sodium or no- salt- added chickpeas, drained
1/2 cup raw almonds
3/4 cup dates
1 apple, cored
1 teaspoon pure vanilla bean powder or alcohol-free vanilla extract
1/4 cup water
2/3 cup old fashioned rolled oats
2/3 cup 100% cacao chocolate chips

Preheat oven to 350 degrees F.

Blend chickpeas, almonds, dates, apple, vanilla and water in a high-powered blender until smooth.

Place in a bowl and mix in oats and chocolate chips.

Drop on a lightly-oiled or parchment-lined baking sheet in 2 tablespoon scoopfuls. Flatten a little with a fork.

Bake for 10 minutes.

Makes 20 cookies

NUTRIENT IQ POINTS: 13 per cookie

CALORIES 211; PROTEIN 6g; CARBOHYDRATES 28g; SUGARS 13g; TOTAL FAT 9.5g; SATURATED FAT 3.2g; CHOLESTEROL 0.3mg; SODIUM 5mg; FIBER 5.8g; BETA-CAROTENE 12ug; VITAMIN C 1mg; CALCIUM 45mg; IRON 3.8mg; FOLATE 49ug; MAGNESIUM 63mg; POTASSIUM 295mg; ZINC 1mg; SELENIUM 2.2ug

REFERENCES

1. Kamal R, Cox C. How Has U.S. Spending on Healthcare Changed Over Time? Peterson-KFF Health System Tracker. December 10, 2018, https://www.healthsystemtracker.org/chart-collection/u-s-spending-healthcare-changed-time/#item-start

2. Biener, A., Cawley, J. & Meyerhoefer, C. J GEN INTERN MED (2017) 32(Suppl 1): 6. https://doi.org/10.1007/s11606-016-3968-8.

3. Duke Medicine. "Health care costs steadily increase with body mass." ScienceDaily. ScienceDaily, 16 December 2013. <www.sciencedaily.com/releases/2013/12/131216142222.htm>.

4. Fryar CD, Carrol MD, Ogden CL. Prevalence of Overweight, Obesity, and Extreme Obesity Among Adults Aged 20 and Over: United States, 1960–1962 Through 2015–2016". National Center for Health Statistics. October2018.

5. Qu Q, Paulose-Rom R, Burt VL, et al. Perscription cholesterol-lowering medication use in adults aged 40 andover.: United States 2003-2012. NCHS Sata Brief #177 December 2014

6. Drake V, Micronutrient Inadequacies in the US Population: an Overview. Linus Pauling Institute Micronutrient Information Center 2018

7. Franz MJ, Van Wormer JJ, Crain AL, et al. Weight-loss outcomes: a systematic review and meta-analysis of weight-loss clinical trials with a minimum 1 year follow up. J Am Diet Assoc. 2007;107(10):1755-1767.

8. Fuhrman J, Sarter B, Glaser D, Acocella S. Changing Perceptions of Hunger on a High Nutrient Density Diet. Nutrition Journal 2010; 9:51.

9. Svendsen M, Blomhoff R, Holme I, Tonstad S. The Effect of an increased intake of vegetables and fruit on weight loss, blood pressure and antioxidant defense in subjects with sleep related breathing disorders. Euro J Clin Nutr. 2007; 61:13011311. Ello-Martin JA, Roe LS, Ledikwe JH, et al. Dietary energy density in the treatment of obesity: a year-long trial comparing two weight loss diets. Am J Clin Nutr. 2007: 85(6):1465-1477. Howard BV, Manson JE, Stefanick ML, et al. Low-fat dietary pattern and weight change over seven years: The Women's Health Initiative Dietary Modification Trial. JAMA. 2006; 295(1):39-49.

10. Halberg O, Johansson O. Cancer Trends during the 20th Century. J Aust Coll Nutr Environ Med 2002; 21(1):3-8

11. Liu RH. Potential Synergy of phytochemicals in cancer prevention: mechanism of action. J Nutr. 2004; 134(12) Suppl):3479S-3485S. Weiss JF, Landauer MR. Protection against ionizing radiation by antioxidant nutrients and phytochemicals. Toxicology 2003; 189(1-2):1-20. Carratu B, Sanzini E. Biologically-active phytochemicals in vegetable food. Ann 1st Super Sanita. 2005; 41(1):7-16

12. Hu FB, Willett WC. Optimal diets for prevention of coronary heart disease. JAMA. 2002 Nov 27; 288(20):2569-2578. Esselstyn CB. Resolving the coronary artery disease epidemic through plant-based nutrition. 2001 Autumn; 4(4): 171-177.

13. Lawton CL, Burley VJ, Wales JK, Blundell JE. Dietary fat and appetite control in obese subjects: weak effects on satiation and satiety. Int J Obes Metab Disord. 1991; 17(7): 409-416. Blundell JE, Halford JC. Regulation of nutrient supply: The brain and appetite control. Proc Nutr Soc. 1994; 53(2): 407418. Stamler J, Dolecek TA. Relation of food and nutrient intakes to body mass on the multiple risk factor intervention trial. Am J Clin Nutr. 1997; 65(1 Suppl): 366s-373s

14. Fontana L, Partridge L, Longo VD. Extending healthy life span from yeast to humans. Science. 2010 Apr 16; 328(5976):321-6.

15. Mattes RD, Donnelly D. Relative Contributions of dietary sodium source. J Am Coll Nutr. 1991 Aug; 10(4): 383-93.

NOTES

_____

_____

_____

FOR MORE INFORMATION, VISIT:

www.DrFuhrman.com

Dr. Fuhrman's official website for information, recipes, supportive services, and products

OR CALL:

800-474-WELL (9355)